D0616565

SPECIAL OFFER FOR HEALTH PROFESSIONALS

We have created a special webinar accompanying this book called *"The Life Cycle of a Successful Practice."*

YOU CAN WATCH IT BY REGISTERING AT
GOEVOMED.COM/LIFECYCLE

WHAT YOU WILL LEARN

- Why the "Functional Micropractice" is the basis for any practice vision?

- Which are the best strategies to drive new patients into your practice?

- What should be your first investments as you grow your practice?

- What structures do you need in place for a scalable practice?

You will hear examples from doctors and health professionals in the field.

We look forward to welcoming you to the webinar!

REGISTER TODAY AT
WWW.GOEVOMED.COM/LIFECYCLE

"Chronic disease is this century's greatest challenge and medicine must adapt to meet it. It is becoming clear that Functional Medicine is a vastly improved operating system for treating chronic disease, but until now there was no road map for physicians to create the new practice model necessary to practice it efficiently. I highly recommend this book to any of my physician colleagues looking to fall back in love with practicing medicine, and given its exquisite timing, this book might just change the world."

— MARK HYMAN, MD, Director,
Cleveland Clinic Center for Functional Medicine

"The leading sources of morbidity, premature mortality, and high costs of care in developed countries around the world— the so-called chronic, non-communicable diseases—persist and progress despite the best conventional treatments, but are eminently preventable, and at times reversible, with lifestyle as medicine. Getting that medicine to go down, and directing medical attention past effects to underlying causes requires new models, such as those elucidated here. James Maskell describes in terms both visionary, and practical, the necessary evolution of medical practice to foster revolutionary improvements in the human condition. I hope many will follow where James is leading."

— DAVID KATZ, MD, President,
American College of Lifestyle Medicine

"With physicians losing faith in industrialized medicine at record speed, a new paradigm is needed to engage both physicians and patients into health creation. The 'Functional Micropractice' is a fascinating concept and will accelerate the movement towards truly integrated healthcare. I recommend this book to any physician colleague."

— DEEPAK CHOPRA, MD, FACP,
Founder of the Chopra Center for Wellbeing

"We are in the midst of a sea change. Medicine, as we know it, is succumbing to the forces of evolution and opportunity is springing from the rubble. Clinicians, debt-saddled, overwhelmed, and burnt out by their conventional training, are learning that they have a choice: They can choose between a deeply fulfilling and financially rewarding experience as a healer or they can punch the clock in an insurance-based mill of a practice. James Maskell is uniquely ordained to help light the path for clinicians to this space of opportunity, self-realization, and connection to the wisdom of holistic and integrative medicine. Visionary, thought leader, and pragmatist, James has created the handbook for how to reclaim your life purpose, and to contribute personally to the most important revolution of our time."

— KELLY BROGAN, MD, Holistic Psychiatrist,
author of *A Mind of Your Own*

"Chronic disease is on the rise. Doctors are disillusioned with their jobs. This is a devastating combination. James masterfully addresses both these areas with aplomb. We have heard about solutions to the chronic disease burden before but there has always been a missing piece. How do doctors first learn these skills and then, most importantly, how do doctors put these ideas into practice in a medical system fast becoming unfit for purpose? For doctors looking to make the switch, this book provides a step by step guide. If you are a frustrated medical professional looking for another way, you have to read this book! The population's health is getting worse—we are devolving. It is time for medicine to evolve."

— RANGAN CHATTERJEE, MD,
Supergeneralist and BBC One's "Doctor in the House"

"We need doctors who love their work and patients who love their doctors again. And we need practitioners who are able to respond intelligently and effectively to the crises going on in our health and healthcare. This new wave that James Maskell presents to us in The Evolution of Medicine offers a healing balm that has the potential to change the tide for us all—and for the better that we so desperately need."

— AVIVA ROMM, MD, Yale Integrative Medicine

"We are living through what will certainly be viewed as an ironic chapter in the history of medicine. As consumers, employers and governments buckle under the financial weight of chronic disease, the system is perversely designed to thwart the efforts of doctors seeking to address the problem for us all. As they seek to invest the time and master the technology required to find and resolve the underlying causes of chronic disease, the system exerts itself against them—pushing them to work faster rather than smarter. In this book, James Maskell offers a practical path forward for the physician champions of the next era of medicine. Amidst the frightening consolidation of primary care, he proposes a much needed avenue to preserve the independent practitioner and realign the value they create in the healthcare economy with the value they are able to capture for themselves and their families."

— TOM BLUE, Chief Strategy Officer,
American Academy of Private Physicians

"The world is changing, and so is medicine. As you probably know, chronic disease is both the largest killer and the largest healthcare expense in the modern world, and medicine as we currently know it is doing a pretty poor job of addressing that. The medicine of the future—the medicine that James Maskell advocates for—will be founded on sound lifestyle principles, and will reinvent the way that providers and patients connect. Connection is the theme here: providers with patients, patients with their own bodies, and all humans with the earth and with each other. I'm excited to support James as he works to design and fertilize a new operating system for creating health. The world has a brighter future because of this book."

— DALLAS HARTWIG,
co-author of *The Whole30* and *It Starts With Food*

"Thank you, James Maskell, for shedding light on our current 'medical industry' and the ill effects of the system on our doctors. James offers us hope and tangible solutions for a better healthcare system where 'health' and 'care' are our top values and priorities for both patients and doctors. Medicine needs a FRESH start and James started a movement, an evolution!"

— ROBERT E. Graham, MD, MPH, ABOIM, FACP

THE
EVOLUTION
OF MEDICINE

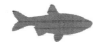

Join the Movement to Solve

Chronic Disease and

Fall Back in Love with Medicine

JAMES MASKELL

THE EVOLUTION OF MEDICINE
Join the Movement to Solve Chronic Disease
and Fall Back in Love with Medicine

ISBN   978-1-61961-509-0 Paperback
       978-1-61961-510-6 Ebook
       978-1-61961-511-3 Audiobook

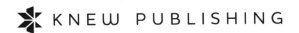 KNEW PUBLISHING

FOR MY DAUGHTER, KALIANA,

AND HER GENERATION, WHO DESPERATELY

NEED OUR HELP

CONTENTS

SYNOPSIS

ONE OF THE CORE findings of this book is that doctors and health professionals are struggling with work-life balance, and understandably have limited time to read long texts. I have distilled this book into the following synopsis so you can quickly determine if it speaks to you. (You're welcome!)

THE STATE OF THE EVOLUTION

The great paleontologist Stephen Jay Gould said that evolution proceeds, not slowly and steadily, but with long periods of little or no change punctuated by intervals of sudden, rapid, and significant shift. If evolution is defined as adapting to one's environment, then medicine is indeed readying for this growth. The medical environment has transformed quickly over the last five decades, with the impressive gains in lifespan and communicable diseases being overshadowed by the rapid growth (and associated massive cost increases) of chronic and noncommunicable diseases (NCDs).

This is not purely an American problem, but America is certainly feeling it harder than others. As of 2016, American healthcare makes up 18.8% of GDP, and although that percentage is the highest in the world by some margin (the average is 6%) the top diagnoses in countries once considered "third world" are not what you might expect: not cholera, typhoid, or TB, but our familiar foes, type 2 diabetes, heart disease, and cancer.

Unlike doctors, I see this issue through a lens of economics, and America's prevalence of chronic disease is intimately linked to huge costs. It is estimated by some to make up as much as 80% of total healthcare costs and is scheduled to cost $47 trillion over the next decade. How high do these numbers have to go before all payers, whether they be regular people, businesses, or even sovereign nations are crushed under these enormous costs? And it's not just the cost of the "medicine." There are often associated costs, such as three full-time helpers needed for each Alzheimer's patient.

The costs of chronic disease are one piece of the puzzle, but what about the doctors themselves? For centuries, becoming a doctor has been a noble calling. Being privy to the innermost details of their patients' lives and deepest vulnerabilities requires levels of care, compassion, and empathy that only certain people are capable of delivering every day, over the course of their entire career.

As you probably already know, the word doctor comes from

the Latin word *docere*, which is synonymous with teacher. I may not be a doctor myself, but I do have a General Certificate of Secondary Education in Latin (earned during a misspent youth and on the very few occasions that my Latin becomes useful I feel it necessary to show it off). The term is fitting, as early physicians were the centers of their community, not only tending to disease but also educating patients in self-care, wellness, and disease prevention. For the majority of the thousands of doctors I've met over the last decade, there was an inner calling to become a doctor, not a conscious choice. The second half of the twentieth century will surely be known in times to come as the "first golden age of medicine" with new wealth, technology, insight, and interventions elevating doctors to an almost God-like stature.

One of the side effects of this huge success was an entrenchment of hierarchy and patriarchy in medicine. The number of non-medical administrators in medicine went through the roof, often bringing with them perverse incentives and a focus away from the patient and toward the balance sheet. Male doctors wrote prescriptions and gave orders to female nurses. Younger doctors deferred to older doctors; few women or minorities were in positions of authority in medicine. Linear thinking was valued as the profession became more and more standardized, and the differential diagnosis reigned supreme.

These side effects went undetected for a while (as is often the case), but in the last decade an awareness has emerged, bringing with it many "symptoms." One such symptom is the number of doctors advising their own children against a career in medicine, sometimes breaking a multigenerational tradition of physician training.

The second symptom is that the level of dissatisfaction among doctors is frighteningly high. A large American physician survey in early 2016 found that 83% of doctors are disillusioned with medicine, and 63% are thinking of quitting in the next two years. But again, this problem isn't just American. Single-payer systems such as the National Health Service in the UK have similar issues, to the point of thousands of doctors going on strike in the last year and leaving medicine at unprecedented rates due to dissatisfaction with conditions, pay, and systemic issues.

According to a recent article, "A 2012 Medscape study found that 46 percent of primary care physicians showed such dissatisfaction with their careers, they wouldn't pursue medicine if they could choose again. Another study, from the Physicians Foundation, found 60 percent of primary care doctors would not recommend a career in medicine. Just six percent described the morale of their colleagues as positive." These statistics from 2012 have only gotten worse since the implementation of the Affordable Care Act (ACA).

For many doctors, the industrialization of medicine means that they aren't truly able to follow their calling. They find themselves unable to help in the ways that they envisioned early on in their training. The love, empathy, and respect they innately have to offer their patients has been lost in the maze of insurance reimbursement forms and revenue targets.

In November 2015, my friend Dr. Pamela Wible's TEDMED talk brought to light another symptom of the emerging dark side of medicine, physician suicide. Many doctors emerge from medical school and residencies with something approximating post-traumatic stress disorder. The long hours, short visits, lack of sleep, high stress environment, fluorescent lights, and convenience food make for personal health crises.

I'm not sure if it was her reading suicide letters from doctors out loud or the pronouncement that one million patients lose their doctor to suicide each year that got me, but something snagged in my heart. For all these reasons and more I have dedicated myself to helping the healers, and I have grand ambitions for scaling this type of aid. If you can help one doctor be more effective, the ripple effect can impact more than 30,000 people. I have nothing but the greatest respect for anyone who chooses this noble path and also has the motivation and resilience to make it through something as grueling as medical school and residency training. This topic surely enrages us all, whichever vantage point you come from. On a recent Functional Forum podcast episode with Dr. Wible, she shared a ray of hope that perhaps this provocative issue will be a catalyst for medicine to really take a deeper look at the negative side effects of its own industrialization. I, for one, hope she is right.

So the real question is: Do you feel me?

Does this resonate with you?

If so, you are in the right place, and thank you for being here.

The good news is this: It isn't all doom and gloom, in fact, quite the opposite.

THE NEW MODEL

The subtitle of this book is "join the movement to solve chronic disease and fall back in love with medicine," and that is exactly the opportunity here before you. Dr. Pamela Wible says that "doctors 'will be in mass exodus' once they learn they can run their practice differently and 'get off the production line.'" This book seeks to be a guide for that journey.

There is a grand convergence afoot, where, for the first time, there is a unique confluence of circumstances through which we can solve not only the problem of chronic disease, but also doctor dissatisfaction.

This elegant solution is akin to the farmers' market revolution in the food system. After decades of a highly industrialized food system, a certain segment of the American population demanded real food directly from the farmer, cutting out all the middlemen and harkening back to a more sustainable, mutually valuable relationship with our food system. As this became more popular, farmers' markets grew in number and popularity. Growing demand brought organization and technology, which led to Community Supported Agriculture (CSAs), and tempered pricing. All of a sudden, Costco is organic, Whole Foods are springing up everywhere, and now startups are emerging to make it easier and more cost effective than ever to get healthy food. I'm definitely not saying the food system is fully repaired by any means, but these are encouraging trends and the same opportunity is available in medicine, as we are still in the early adopter phase. In this book we will share stories of doctors I consider the founding fathers of this medical evolution, taking up the challenge and sharing best practices so you can learn from their mistakes.

If you are reading this book before 2020, you can be one of the early adopters of a new operating system for medicine, designed from the ground up to be effective for chronic disease. You can then deliver this upgraded version of primary care, what some have called "supergeneralism" directly to your community, cutting out the middleman. Side effects may include starting to live the stress-free lives you would probably like to prescribe to your patients.

The other benefit to this plan to evolve medicine is that doctors can become part owners of the revolution, and not just the mid-level employees or henchmen. By engaging the ingenuity of the community and using technology to share best practices amongst clinician-entrepreneurs, we can not only provide a structure for you to fall back in love with medicine but also set a set a model for the rest of the world to follow.

SERVING THE COMMUNITY

To solve chronic disease, we need medicine delivered to where people actually are, in their communities. We need only look to the Blue Zones (five places on the planet with most centenarians and lowest levels of chronic disease) to see that they don't have access to a lot of novel, expensive medical technology, but they make amazing use of the fundamental technologies of health creation: healthy food, strong communities, low stress, and regular exercise.

In his book *The Daniel Plan,* Dr. Mark Hyman shared this incredible story of his work at the Saddleback Church, where, with the support of their celebrity pastor Rick Warren, the church's population of 15,000 lost a combined 250,000 pounds and dozens of diagnoses by taking full advantage of the incredible power of community. Dan Buettner's efforts to bring the learnings of the Blue Zones to America has led to 41% reductions in cost through similar strategies.

In this book, we are going to examine the opportunity for doctors and other health professionals to build community micropractices, serving their practice members directly through a combination of in-person visits and telemedicine. These new practice models are popping up where people actually are: co-working spaces, gyms, corporate campuses, CrossFit boxes, community centers, strip malls, and churches. With the low overhead of these nontraditional medical settings, plus the focus on the things that patients really want (like more time with the doctor and thoughtful use of technology), these practices are flourishing all over the country.

In the first half of this book, we will dive deeply into this new model—not only the specifics of the clinical operating system but also the thinking process behind it. We will learn lessons from the earliest adopters on the cutting edge of medical evolution, the typical challenges and ways they overcame them. We will show you how clinician-entrepreneurs have tailored the model to their patient populations and zip codes, focusing on successful strategies to deliver this care beyond its current demographics, whom my friend Dr. Robin Berzin refers to as the "very rich, very sick and very green."

In the second half of the book, we will share the best practices for dealing with some of the common pitfalls in building this type of practice, focusing on efficiency. If you are going to offer a higher quality of care to your patients, spending more time with them and helping to get to the root cause of their issues, there will not be enough doctor's hours to go around for everyone who needs this kind of care. As a result, sensible use of provider teams, group and community structures, and best-in-category technologies will allow you to serve patients at the highest level.

At the end of the book, we will also curate some simple next steps for any physicians interested in joining this movement to solve chronic disease and fall back in love with medicine.

WHY SHOULD YOU LISTEN TO ME?

This is one of the biggest questions I get from people when I tell them what I do: If you aren't a doctor or health professional, why do they listen to you?

For the last eleven years I've been passionately involved in this work. My first job was running a clinic that was designed to be a new model for the delivery of primary care. It was housed in a day spa in rural Georgia and remains one of the best-run practices I have ever seen.

Since then, I've had the opportunity to meet with and listen to thousands of doctors and health professionals, first, through my job as a sales representative, where I traveled to every small town from Virginia to Maine. Following that, I owned and ran a practice management company and a practice marketing company, all serving the modern doctor.

In 2014, I co-founded Evolution of Medicine. Over the last few years, we built and hosted over 30 episodes of the first live "medutainment" show for health professionals, which is seen by over 10,000 health professionals each month and in over 200 worldwide meet-up groups across six continents. We have created two-week-long digital summits with over 100,000 attendees, interviewed hundreds of leading doctors and technology entrepreneurs for our Functional Forum podcast, and my partner has personally spoken to thousands of doctors. To say we have a good overview of the pulse of the industry would be a massive understatement.

We have already helped dozens of doctors take the leap toward owning their own community micropractice. Many of them have built larger practices on that solid foundation. Our vision for solving chronic disease is a nationwide network of these practices, all physician-owned and operating independently. Our goals with this book are to reduce the barriers to entry for all health professionals to either start or join one of these practices, working together achieve the mission.

Anyone familiar with Joseph Campbell's work might recognize that this book is a classic hero's journey—a journey for health professionals to practice a type of medicine relevant to today's disease, and a journey to fall back in love with medicine. The greatest test will be the practicalities of running the private practice, but the heroes who have already trodden the path will share what they have learned along the way to guide your journey.

In fact, we will go deeper into this story, as the ultimate hero in true, lasting, and meaningful healthcare reform are the patients, and so an intimate knowledge and personal experience of this framework will leave you in good stead to be an effective guide for them.

Thank you for being with me on this journey.

CHAPTER ONE

A NEW MODEL

You never change things by fighting the existing reality.
To change something, build a new model that makes the
existing model obsolete.

— R. BUCKMINSTER FULLER

W HEN DR. RANGAN CHATTERJEE describes the moment
he knew, his eyes are full of tears. He explains to the
audience at TEDxLiverpool that he and his wife were on vaca-
tion when she cried out to him that their six-month-old baby
was immobile. Thinking the baby was choking, Dr. Chatterjee
tried to clear his airway, but it didn't work. They rushed the
child to the hospital, where they found he had a hypo-calce-
mic convulsion due to a vitamin D deficiency. "A preventable
deficiency," Dr. Chatterjee says. The baby needed intravenous
calcium and a high dose of vitamin D to save him.

Although he had fourteen years of medical training, Dr. Chatterjee felt wholly unequipped. Being unable to detect a preventable condition in his own child caused him to rethink his entire practice.

For Dr. Jeffrey Gladd, it was his own health. He was fifty pounds overweight, his wife had just given birth to their second child, he took SSRIs to treat panic attacks, and he saw thirty to forty patients per day in the family practice office where he worked. Though he was a young dad and newly-minted doctor, he frequently felt tired and sick. "Not only was my physical health not great," he said, "but my career health wasn't all that great either."

If you have ever seen Dr. Gladd lecture, then you have met his alter ego, Fat Jeff. One of the first slides he shows at presentations is a picture of him in 2005, with his t-shirt stretched around his waistline and soft rolls of skin that frame his face and neck. It was around this time that Dr. Gladd started questioning his life and career. He felt as sick as the people he treated each day.

"There's got to be a different way than this," he said. "I'm unhealthy, my patients are unhealthy, they're looking to me to make them healthy, but I'm no different than them. I don't have the answers."

Over the last eleven years, I've personally met thousands of physicians, nurses, and other health professionals whose stories echo Dr. Chatterjee's and Dr. Gladd's. Across the healthcare industry, doctors are overworked and overtaxed, and the current framework is leading to a pervading sense of dis-ease and unease among healthcare professionals—which may manifest as obesity, anxiety, depression, fatigue, or chronic illness. While some start to question the effectiveness of their practice when they become ill, others are driven to make a shift when a loved one falls ill—like a parent, spouse, sibling, or child. Whatever the reason, this call to adventure is the beginning of the "Hero's Journey," outlined in Joseph Campbell's book by the same name.

What prompted both Dr. Gladd and Dr. Chatterjee to change was an underlying feeling of discontent. Many doctors who go into medicine with the intention of helping and healing often begin to sense that there's something wrong, and that things aren't quite adding up. For some, the presence of a McDonald's or Burger King in the hospital cafeteria sends mixed messages about health, diet, and well-being. Other doctors become uncomfortable treating chronic diseases with more and more prescriptions—sometimes to treat the side effects of others—but without seeing any real improvement or a plan for long-term resolution. What doctors notice in and around hospitals and clinics is a lack of congruence between the way medicine is practiced and what they know to be healthy, which is a cause for concern.

One fundamental question many doctors on this path have considered is, "Can my patients actually get healthier through

the interventions I'm delivering?" Though prescriptions, surgeries, and treatments can 'cure disease,' they aren't designed
to be creating health. Unfortunately, creating health isn't a
part of the coursework of most medical programs, and a standard practice does not provide a framework to help patients
make changes. Few are taught how to deal with the epidemics
of lifestyle-driven chronic disease. They have the tools to deal
with downstream factors—like a diabetic neuropathy or insulin resistance—but not upstream factors—like the impact of
nutrition and lifestyle on blood sugar. As Dr. Chatterjee points
out, with type 2 diabetes, high blood sugar is a symptom, not
the root cause. In order to reverse a chronic disease, we need
to address those root causes.

Dr. Chatterjee and Dr. Gladd's revelations that "there has to be
a better way" prompted them to explore other avenues. They
knew that they couldn't get where they wanted to go within
the current framework. The good news is there is another
way, and, like these heroic doctors, we can all heed the call
to adventure.

Good news: The timing couldn't be better. We are living during
a time of a grand convergence in medicine, where many different factors are all pointing us toward a new paradigm for
creating health. The biggest question is: Where shall we start?

We first see this convergence emerging from Silicon Valley.
New systems, like wearable technology with sleep and activity trackers, are allowing people to take health into their

own hands by tracking their data. Technology has empowered people with access to information so that they might better understand how to create health in themselves. These technologies are evolving to monitor factors that have previously only been medical—blood pressure, blood sugar, and heart rate variability, among others. There's a number on their watch, and people want to learn how to improve it.

The promise of technology doesn't end there by any means. There's a genomic revolution happening, where we can now sequence genes quickly and repeatedly and see how behaviors affect the expression of these genes, both at the most minute level and at the macro level. These technologies are following Moore's Law perfectly, with costs falling and capacity rising exponentially. The emerging field of epigenetics, piggybacking on the genomic revolution, is catalyzing a shift in understanding of how to create health. The study of inheritable changes in gene expression has led to the idea that health outcomes are not only a result of genetics per se, but also heavily influenced by the environment.

We are living in times of second generation automation and communication systems that afford patients more ease in scheduling and connectivity, as well as systems that help a doctor stay up-to-date on a patient's care and treatment. Telemedicine is a prime example of this, being used to empower healthcare, from major cities to rural areas, and everywhere in between. At this exact moment in time, truly useful technologies are arriving to help significantly lower the costs of delivering great care and make the vision of running a whole practice off a single laptop a reality.

We're also seeing a shift in which environmental and evolutionary concepts are being applied to medicine. How did we evolve to create resilient systems to create health?

Since the completion of the Human Microbiome Project in 2011 and the subsequent deluge of new science, the importance of gut bacteria to health has turned conventional medicine on its head when it comes to our primary foes of 20th century medicine, the germ. Patients and doctors alike are learning in real time that bacteria and other microbes are not only beneficial when they're in balance, but they affect every organ and system in the body, from our brains to our joints. Dr. Alessio Fasano's work as a pediatric gastroenterologist and researcher at Harvard has found that the rising issue of autoimmune diseases is related not only to the integrity of the gut and microbiome but also to triggers from our environment.

These aren't the only examples of evolutionary concepts entering the health ecosystem. The paleo diet has become a massive trend in America and worldwide, where participants consider a fundamental question: What were we evolved to eat? Today's industrialized food system includes a lot of processed ingredients and elements that aren't found in nature. It has caused people to ask whether the "evolutionary mismatch" between what we used to eat and what we now eat has led to the rise in chronic disease. It's also becoming clear that one size doesn't fit all.

But how is all of this new information affecting consumer behavior? A 2016 study for the National Center for Complementary and Integrative Health (NCCIH) showed that, in 2012, Americans spent $30.2 billion out-of-pocket on a wide range of complementary health approaches. That included herbal supplements, acupuncture, massage therapy, meditation, chiropractic, and yoga. Within that $30.2 billion, $12.8 billion was spent on natural product supplements alone, which was one-quarter of the amount spent out-of-pocket on prescription drugs. Concepts that were once considered trends or fads are now commonly accepted practices or industries, such as gyms, juice bars, and yoga studios, among others. All of this is happening for the most part quite separately from the practice of medicine.

All of these occurrences clearly point to the need for a new way to engage patients. Modern medicine needs to figure out how to treat patients individually, to spend time with them, and stimulate and support behavioral changes that lead to better health outcomes. We need a system that considers the root causes, as opposed to simply treating the symptoms. We need to help create health, and one way to do that is to seek places where this is already happening.

In Dan Buettner's book, *The Blue Zones,* the author looks at places in the world where residents live long, healthy lives that are free from chronic disease. The locations he studied were Loma Linda, California; Nicoya, Costa Rica; Icaria, Greece; Sardinia, Italy; and Okinawa, Japan. These regions were not well connected to hospitals or systems of Western medicine, yet the residents lived to be a hundred because their lifestyles were conducive to good health, and they had communities that supported these practices.

Here is the fundamental point: We can't create a "Blue Zone" with conventional medicine—that is, prescription drugs and surgeries alone will not help people lead healthy lives into their tenth decade. Modern medicine does not create health; it treats symptoms and acute disease. If we want to cure chronic disease and move toward cultivating Blue Zones in our communities, we need to adopt a new framework.

What would be the features of this new framework? Dr. Eric Topol, author of *The Creative Destruction of Medicine,* sums up it up succinctly: "An individualistic ideology for how medicine goes forward will not happen soon enough without the people who have the greatest stake—the individuals—to be fully participatory. There will be titanic changes ahead—medicine can and will be rebooted and reinvented one individual at a time."

In Silicon Valley medical circles, like Singularity University's FutureMed conference led by Dr. Daniel Kraft, the prevailing framework for this new model is described as "P4 Medicine," which was conceived by Dr. Leroy Hood, founder of the Institute for Systems Biology.

The four Ps in question are *predictive, preventive, personalized*, and *participatory*. Each one of these gives a fascinating insight into the future of medicine. The first three Ps speak to a new era of technology-enabled healthcare, the final one a definitive shift in the most important person in a medical relationship.

Good examples of predictive medicine can be seen in areas as diverse as clinical lab testing to subtle changes in wearable data, even accessed from across the world. One of the leading voices in this conversation is Dr. Russell Jaffe, who shared at a recent event the eight basic tests he recommends for practicing effective, predictive medicine on every patient, and going upstream to reduce costs. These include the following tests, and for each there are healthy predictive ranges: Hemoglobin A1c, C-Reactive Protein, Homocysteine, Lymphocyte Response Assay, Urine pH, Vitamin D, Omega 3:6 EFA Ratio, and 8-Oxo-Guanine. It is clear that as we start to understand chronic disease as a journey, not as an event, there are obvious markers that tell us patients are moving along that path before they hit the required standard for a differential diagnosis.

A truly preventive medical system would use these signals for both primary and secondary prevention. As the first Chinese medical text says, "The superior doctor prevents sickness; the mediocre doctor attends to impending sickness; the inferior doctor treats actual sickness."

Personalized medicine has been available for a while but typically only to the very rich. Twentieth-century science was solely focused on "what is the most effective treatment for the average human?" It is now clear that there not a lot of "average humans" walking the planet, and that our genetics, microbiomes and exposomes (the total sum of our environmental exposures over our lifetimes) are so diverse and unique that personalization is critical to effectively creating health. Technology is arriving just in time to make that a reality for all.

The final P, participatory, can be enabled by technology but will require deeper engagement for most people. A patient-centered medical model empowers patients to participate in their own care. This is a totally new era for medicine, because in acute disease, participation was not required by the patient. The medicine was done *to* them. This is leading to new skill sets being needed in medicine, seen in the massive rise of coaches—nurse coaches, health coaches, diabetes coaches. Coaching has never before been a part of medicine; it was gleaned from business. But as the need for behavior change becomes more obvious, this is a new key player in the healthcare ecosystem.

The P4 approach is the most comprehensive concept for the new paradigm in medicine, showing a new way to engage patients, to treat people individually, to take time with them, and to motivate them to make behavior and lifestyle changes that will lead to better health outcomes and, ideally, new Blue Zones.

The real question then becomes something we haven't really considered. How do we (re)train an army of new providers to deliver P4 Medicine? How can we best accelerate this evolution of medicine? The truth is, we need a fully realized system for delivering the promise of P4 Medicine. We need a common language for all providers, from specialists to generalists to the new army of health coaches, to understand each patient as an individual and work together to empower each one to achieve health.

For the first five years of my new career in America, I was looking for that fully realized system. I was exposed to lifestyle medicine, holistic medicine, naturopathic medicine, and integrative medicine. They all had the potential to be part of the solution. They were all grounded in principles of health creation and treating the individual and not the disease, and when looked at from 30,000 feet are fundamentally similar, but there are two elephants in the room that compromise their ability to be the new system: language and reproducibility.

The language issue speaks for itself. I bet most reading this would struggle to pick apart the definitions of the words used above. Most providers who practice medicine with those names will tell you that the practice of it is an art and a science, which is totally awesome, until you think about scaling up. How many people can shadow famed Scripps Cardiologist Dr. Mimi Guarneri at once, or apprentice with Dr. David Katz at Yale?

In 2010 I attended my first Integrative Health Symposium in New York City and had the opportunity to sit in on a few lectures by some of the leading lights in an emerging field of functional medicine, including its "Founding Father" Dr. Jeffrey Bland and its "Prodigal Son" Dr. Mark Hyman. What struck me straight away was that functional medicine had the opportunity to be the bridge between Western medicine and integrative medicine for two main reasons: language and reproducibility.

By definition, functional medicine addresses the underlying causes of disease using a systems-oriented approach to engage both patient and practitioner through a therapeutic partnership. It's an evolution of the practice of medicine that best addresses the healthcare needs of the 21st century by shifting the traditional disease-centered focus of medical practice to a more patient-centered approach.

Now, I have to at this juncture offer a disclaimer. Several of the doctors I have mentioned in this book do not refer to what they do as "functional medicine." Dr. Jeffrey Gladd practices integrative medicine, Dr. Chatterjee refers to it (at least when he's on TV) as lifestyle medicine. Dr. Dean Ornish will be horrified to hear me referring to his work as functional medicine (even though he is a previous recipient of the Linus Pauling Award for outstanding achievement in Functional Medicine). Other terms used in the past are holistic medicine, complementary medicine, and alternative medicine, the latter of which almost seems offensive at this point. Alternative to what, exactly? But there are three main reasons why, for the rest of this book, I will refer to it as functional medicine.

First, using this term will make it easier on you, the reader. We want to keep this as clearly defined as possible, and I know the verbiage makes people uncomfortable. Second, we have sought to be a bridge, through our content and meet-ups, for these providers to connect in person and realize that 90% of what they do is completely congruent, and we are stronger together than siloed. Third, and most importantly, I think of it in terms of scale. The most important thing that functional medicine has going for it is a reproducible system to train new clinicians on how to deliver truly predictive, preventive, personalized, and participatory medicine.

Functional medicine efficiently organizes the combination of standard of care and nonstandard of care modalities that are a feature of integrative medicine, helping clinicians to prioritize interventions for the individual in front of them. It is definitely based in lifestyle medicine, so much so that the 2016 Annual Conference of the Institute for Functional Medicine was focused clearly on lifestyle medicine. It has things in common with naturopathic medicine, like treating the whole person, the doctor as teacher, and the concept of the "therapeutic order"—using the least costly and least invasive modalities first. Anyone concerned with the cost trajectory of healthcare can see the obvious merit in this.

Functional medicine serves as an operating system for health creation that allows doctors to individuate the approach, which is currently the only repeatable, reproducible, and consistent way to create health that is widely practiced today.

Other styles of medicine don't have a repeatable system to train a lot of doctors, and we need a reproducible model to help a new army of doctors and other clinicians deliver more effective, consistent care in their communities.

At the center of this operating system is the Functional Medicine Matrix, providing the consistent framework to deliver functional medicine. With this as a guide, doctors uncover not only a comprehensive timeline of the patient's health but also the predisposing factors (antecedents), precipitating events (triggers), and ongoing contributors (mediators) of a patient's chronic health problem. It's a systematic, scientific, and reproducible way to understand a patient.

There are a couple of other factors that make functional medicine a great bet for the future of chronic care. First and foremost, one of the most storied medical organizations in the world is making the same bet.

The Cleveland Clinic, consistently rated one of the top five hospitals in the country, opened the Center for Functional Medicine in collaboration with the Institute for Functional Medicine (IFM) in October 2014. The clinic is led by Dr. Mark Hyman, founder of The UltraWellness Center and a ten-time *New York Times* best-selling author. He actually announced the collaboration to the practitioner community on the fourth episode of our show, the Functional Forum (which also happened to feature Dr. Gladd).

Since it opened, the center has been oversubscribed, with more people signing up than it can handle, and in 2016, it was expanded to 18,000 square feet. The Cleveland Clinic always wants to be on the cutting edge of medicine, and they're betting that functional medicine is the operating system for the future of chronic care. This is not just a clinical effort; they are also doing massive research on outcomes data for a range of chronic conditions, and the early signs are very promising. If I were to look into my crystal ball, I would predict that in 2018, at the exact moment when the outcomes studies arrive from the Cleveland Clinic for proving better outcomes at lower cost, the majority of insurance carriers move fully across to outcome-based payments. That will be quite the convergence.

For physicians who want to apply functional medicine ideas in their practice but are concerned about what their colleagues will think, the prestige of the Cleveland Clinic matters, as does its high demand from patients, and the satisfaction of patient and provider alike. In 2016, for the first time, over one million potential patients will head to the Institute for Functional Medicine's "Practitioner Finder" page.

Another huge asset for functional medicine comes from the technology world. Up until 2015, administering functional medicine was a time-intensive, paper-based system, but as you will see in Chapter 7, we now have a technology to digitize and standardize this process. This allows the practice of functional medicine to be much more efficient and adds to our ability as a movement to track outcomes across multiple clinics and prove the effectiveness and efficiency of the new paradigm.

Unlike most medications, the side effects of practicing this type of care are beneficial. A recent survey of functional medicine practitioners showed that most of them wanted to keep practicing beyond their 75th birthday, a sure sign that these doctors were hugely fulfilled by practicing medicine in this way.

On our very first Functional Forum, Dr. Kelly Brogan asked the group, "How many of you love your job?" Most of the hands went up. This is in stark contrast to the plight of the average physician, who is sick and tired of industrialized medicine and looking for a way out.

The quotation at the start of this chapter from Bucky Fuller has been on my e-mail signature for three years: "You never change things by fighting the existing reality. To change something, build a new model that makes the existing model obsolete." It is clear to me that functional medicine is the new model that will make the existing model obsolete. If we can go upstream and deal with the causes of chronic disease at the source, we can fulfill the ultimate reality.

Dr. Jeffrey Gladd insisted that there had to be a better way. He started paying attention to nutrition, something he admitted to knowing little about, despite his medical training, and he lost fifty pounds. He got off medication and ultimately realized that his work as a doctor wasn't helping in the way he had hoped. Instead of curing, he felt he was "prolonging and suppressing disease." Wanting to address this, he studied functional medicine, learning how to weave it into his current practice.

He serves as a great example of what can happen when an individual embraces functional medicine before it's endorsed by large health systems, hospitals, or clinics, and now, more than ever, there are resources available to take control and start a "functional micropractice." These practices are popping up all over, from Dr. Gladd's home in Fort Wayne, Indiana to Cairo, Egypt, and the movement is accelerating.

However, Dr. Gladd's path wasn't always paved with success and acceptance. Before science caught up to him, the ideas underpinning this new paradigm were initially considered quackery—one of a few reasons why doctors may resist the call to functional medicine.

QUESTION: *What do you truly love about medicine? What got you into medicine?*

ACTION: *Write your story. Compare what you envisioned you'd be doing to what you're doing now.*

CHAPTER TWO

FACING YOUR FEARS

Everything you've ever wanted is on the other side of fear.
— GEORGE W. ADDAIR, founder, Omega Vector

T HERE ARE PLENTY OF places you can go on the Internet to "prove" that I am wrong. There are many blogs and resource centers that will tell you functional medicine is quackery, and this is just better marketing of unsubstantiated claims. What I hope to show you in this chapter is that science is evolving to support the basis of this new paradigm, and although your feelings and fears are justified, it might not be serving you to be governed by them.

I'm sure if you went through medical school you are aware of the adage often shared in the first class: "50% of what you learn here will turn out not to be true; you just have to work out which 50%." You might also be aware of the new science suggesting that it takes, on average, seventeen years for new clinical information to be practiced widely in medicine. Let's see how this plays out in one particular topic that has been at the center of this argument: toxins.

For decades, naturopathic doctors have been ridiculed for a foundational principle of their medical paradigm that toxins can and do contribute to disease. September 2015 marked a significant shift in the mainstream acceptance of this idea. First, the International Federation of Gynecology and Obstetrics (FIGO) became the first global reproductive health organization to take a stand on human exposure to toxic chemicals. Second, the Endocrine Society did a comprehensive review of the scientific literature and determined that many of the endocrine disrupting chemicals in our environment—from persistent organic pollutants to bisphenol A to pesticides to phthalates—not only harm those exposed to them but also are passed between generations, with a particularly negative impact on infants. This birthed a new term: transgenerational epigenetics.

It may seem obvious to anyone who has seen the deformed grandchildren of the Vietnamese people the US Armed Forces sprayed with Agent Orange during the Vietnam War, but this is happening in much more subtle ways with a broader spectrum of impact. Over the last few years there have been countless studies on a wide range of toxic compounds showing a similar pattern of degradation to our environment. The effects are subtle at first, then get compounded over time as the natural detoxification systems break down and then eventually show themselves as symptoms. The first coal plant in Beijing didn't disrupt the lives of its citizens, but a hundred years later, you can't see your hand in front of your face, and the population is becoming chronically ill at record speed.

Situations like the Flint, Michigan drinking water crisis or the well-publicized reports linking lead exposure to violent crime only separate the populace who are reading about it in the news from doctors who insist this isn't a problem. After all, what tools do you have to offer if this is truly a cause of dysfunction?

Another topic that was a tipping point for me to see the value of functional medicine was the microbiome. My interest was piqued after I attended a lecture by Dr. Robert Rountree at the American College for Advancement in Medicine (ACAM) conference in 2012. Before that, the medical literature on the microbiome was few and far between, even though naturopathic doctors had been touting the symbiotic role of microbes inside us more than a century before. In 1915, Benedict Lust said, "We believe that germs and microbes should be looked upon as beneficent workers instead of enemies to human health." Yet contemporary physicians believed that all germs were bad and aimed to kill as many as possible, ignoring any potential fallout. Now, we understand from the Human Micro-biome Project that more than 99% of bacteria are good for us, regulating our digestion, metabolism, and immunity. Instead of trying to destroy every last one, we're now aiming to create a good synergistic relationship between the person and the microbes within them. We've also learned that the microbiome, or the microorganisms in a specific environment, can affect all different types of diseases—type 2 diabetes, heart disease, joint issues, mental health, and other systems of the body that aren't related to the gut itself.

How could that be, when there's just one major organ inside the body with microbes, the gut? The only way to understand it is through functional medicine, which sees the body through an ecological point of view. Instead of isolating organs or sys-tems, we consider the entire body along with the antecedents, triggers, and mediators.

Dr. Leo Galland, one of the founders of functional medicine, said at the Evolution of Medicine Summit in 2014 that "We are humans, yes, but we are really ecological systems. The real importance of this in the future of medicine is the recogni-tion that it may be possible to treat people and treat illness by addressing the ecology of the human being rather than just attempting to suppress the disease." Treating the body through this framework is a completely different paradigm.

Another topic in this vein is the "leaky gut." Ever since Dr. Leo Galland came up with the concept of leaky gut twenty-five years ago, he was dismissed in mainstream medical circles as a quack. Just like toxins, anything that didn't fit within the accepted paradigm of disease was relegated to quackery.

Quack.

Quackery.

This term is almost onomatopoeic at this stage. How does it make you feel when you say it to yourself?

In the last five years we have seen the mainstream acceptance of leaky gut syndrome in medical journals, as well as other terms and concepts Dr. Galland used that were once dismissed, such as gut dysbiosis and patient-centered care. Educated at NYU-Bellevue Medical Center in New York, Dr. Galland became "disillusioned with the mythology of modern medicine" in the 1970s—namely, how conventional medicine treated the disease but not the individual. Doctors like him are now seen as true pioneers, looking beyond the dogma and learning through treating patients and sharing his findings with a small cohort of other doctors who were seeing the same things. They endured the ridicule of a whole profession that they love, and they have the humility to continue to help people. These are the pioneers who helped create the Functional Medicine Matrix and who have created the opportunity for those of us in the next era.

Many physicians looking to make the switch to functional medicine are afraid of failure. They're afraid of being ridiculed by their peers and colleagues, of being seen as foolish, and especially of being seen as a quack. About five years ago I met with a functional medicine doctor whose husband was a dermatologist. He personally witnessed patients getting better from the care of his wife, even seeing the reversal of chronic skin conditions. He was aware of the studies showing a link between the gut microbiome and skin health and was looking for an edge to keep his practice full and thriving. When I mentioned that every integrative (insert any specialty from dentist to rheumatologist) or physician I knew was booked solid, he insisted that he wouldn't go in that direction, for fear of losing standing among his peers in the dermatology community. This is a story I've told a number of times over the last five years, and I'm happy to report that the tide has turned. This dermatologist is now trained in functional medicine and adding integrative services to his practice.

There's a huge amount of vulnerability that comes with changing careers, or even viewpoints, and creating a new structure of medicine. Many fear that they'll get it wrong—write the wrong prescription or misdiagnose a patient. Some fear that additional training will be too costly or time-consuming. Most feel embarrassed to admit that their extensive medical training may not have fully equipped them to create health.

Doctors are often afraid to transition to functional medicine because they are told throughout medical school to conform to a standard, accepted model. In the 1980s, the American Medical Association (AMA) code of ethics forbade doctors to associate with "unscientific" practitioners, particularly chiropractors. This led to a federal antitrust lawsuit by chiropractors against the AMA, which the chiropractors won in the Supreme Court in 1987. Still, doctors are being told that chiropractic care is worthless. Old paradigms die hard in medicine, but the new AMA code of ethics now says doctors "shall be free to choose whom to serve, with whom to associate, and the environment in which to provide medical services."

Despite this freedom, doctors often dismiss the value of integrative practitioners, even if patients are seeing strong or positive results. It's hard to overcome years of training and conditioning, as well as the hierarchical nature of the industry. It's understandably hard to go against the established system, and it often requires that doctors face the unpleasant truth that many of the things they've been taught were incorrect or incomplete. Even though doctors are warned in medical school, "50% of what you learn here will turn out not to be true; you just have to work out which 50%," they're afraid to question the status quo.

Heeding the call takes courage and humility. Doctors are held in high esteem in our society and are thought to know everything. In order to become a doctor, one has to receive top marks in school, attend a good university, and land a residency. The education of a doctor is grueling, and more and more doctors, including Dr. Pamela Wible, describe it as a traumatic event with symptoms consistent with post-traumatic stress disorder.

If patient care isn't a good enough reason to transition to functional medicine, there's the issue of physician health. Rates of heart attacks and suicide are significantly higher than those of other professions. In Dr. Wible's captivating TEDMED talk in 2015, she states that over one million patients lose their doctor to physician suicide each year. The level of dissatisfaction among doctors is frighteningly high, with one survey finding that 83% of doctors were disillusioned with medicine and 63% considered or planned quitting in the following two years. The problem isn't reserved for the US system—the National Health Service in the UK has similar issues, with doctors going on strike and leaving medicine altogether at unprecedented rates. In the developed world, working conditions for doctors are poor in terms of job satisfaction. Most doctors go into medicine hoping to make a difference, but the system is structured in a way that often defeats them—pressured to see more patients, they feel like they're providing less care. The system is not structured to provide empathy or fulfill a doctor's desire to help and heal. It's hard to imagine anyone providing adequate patient care when they aren't even feeling their best.

Once employed, they become the go-to person for every question—administrators, nurses, patients, and friends and family. To admit that their approach to creating health might be inaccurate or incomplete opens up the possibility of the unknown. If what we've been taught isn't working, then what will?

The fear of the unknown is really common when doctors contemplate the shift to functional medicine. Recognizing that something's not right, they often bounce ideas off colleagues. If they were all educated in the same system, then they'll all possess the same answers, and many will convince each other that it's a bad idea or it won't work. Even industry conferences held outside the parameters of the hospital or clinic seek only to prove and reiterate the established knowledge—which is often dominated by conventional and conservative approaches and/or funded by special-interest groups.

None of us wants to feel like we don't have the answers, especially in our chosen field, having devoted years of our life to the pursuit of that knowledge. Many in the field of functional medicine have said that the only reason they got over their fear was because they had to—a health crisis, theirs or a loved one's, led them to make the shift.

Physicians still resist making the switch because of some common misperceptions. Functional medicine was seen as a system that needed doctors to spend a lot of time with people and patients. Up until now, it wasn't worked out into a repeatable system or properly researched to demonstrate outcomes and economic feasibility. Functional medicine has also been mainly delivered in private practice, so doctors have to build the skills of an entrepreneur, business owner, manager, and marketer, and there can be a steep learning curve and associated training costs that keep people from participating.

Perhaps the biggest misperception that keeps doctors from making the switch is that they assume they need a huge practice, with big overhead and a lot of space. If a physician trained in a hospital and worked only inside a major health system or large clinic, then they'll assume that it's the only way to deliver medicine.

Luckily, this too is changing. People who have already implemented functional medicine are starting to communicate best practices so that the learning curve is significantly shorter. Functional medicine is now easily repeatable and reproducible. By starting small and scaling up over time, "functional micropractices" can be low overhead. New technologies like telemedicine and patient tracking allow a micropractice to be run out of a single-room office, and they are popping up in nontraditional medical settings like community centers, co-working spaces, gyms, CrossFits, and churches.

Gone are the days where the only value delivered by a practice is the care of the main doctor. Instead, doctors can create value by creating a team of synergistic providers, being available via telemedicine, sending automated e-mail education campaigns, connecting patients to coaches or accountability groups for individuals with the same ailments. There is a lot of opportunity to add value outside the billable hours of the main physician.

Another misconception is that you have to know everything about functional medicine before you can build a functional medicine practice. Since you're already trained as a clinician, you only have to know enough to get your functional medicine practice started, and the rest will follow. Although doctors are often taught that they have to know everything, the most important part of functional medicine isn't knowing but just being there—listening to people, having empathy, and curating resources. The barriers to entry are pretty low.

In Dr. Leo Galland's case, he slowly integrated functional medicine into his practice, calling patients to follow up and ask what steps they were taking to maintain their health. Dr. Jeffrey Gladd said he made the shift by asking questions: "Here I am, in my busy primary care [practice], getting ready to write a prescription for a statin and doubling the dose of insulin, and I just stopped and started looking at patients and saying, 'What are you eating? Tell me about your relationships. Tell me about stress. Tell me about sleep.'"

Many doctors who transition into functional medicine do so gradually. Since they have a full-time job they can't or don't want to leave, they'll devote one day a week to a functional practice, starting in a small office or community setting. This way, there's low overhead, and they can start small. Instead of worrying about having a full client list, they can focus on a few people and grow with word-of-mouth referrals. This is a great way to titrate their way across until they're all in.

Since many have already taken steps into the unknown, we have their wisdom and resources to learn from. If nothing else, over the last three years, the Evolution of Medicine has sought to be a central focal point for this conversation.

What will it take for the majority of family medicine, primary care, and specialty doctors to come and learn the principles of health creation and incorporate functional medicine?

To answer this question, I lean on the work of one of the greatest social theorists of his generation, Mark Granovetter, whose model to understand the behavior of groups is called the "Threshold Model of Collective Behavior." Your threshold is the number of people that would have to do something in order for you to join in, and for each of us the threshold is different. Unlike beliefs, which are internal things you hold in your head and your heart, thresholds are external, a form of peer pressure. My interpretation is that thresholds have artificially suppressed the masses from switching, but the same forces will massively increase the migration over the coming decade—what Malcolm Gladwell calls "the tipping point." Through this model of collective behavior, we can see how the communities surrounding us affects our behaviors and choices.

QUESTION: *What is your biggest frustration about practicing medicine?*

ACTION: *Make a "not to-do list" of things you no longer want to do.*

CHAPTER THREE

TURNING TO THE COMMUNITY

"Community is the guru of the future."

— THICH NHAT HANH

INSTEAD OF BUILDING A physical practice before seeing patients, Dr. Pamela Wible first went to the community—her would-be patients—to hear what they had to say. After years of practice of assembly-line medicine, she was burned out. Like Dr. Gladd, she felt that there had to be a better way, but wasn't sure what that looked like. She invited members of the community to a town hall meeting in Eugene, Oregon, where they discussed what the ideal medical clinic might look like from the patient's perspective.

What did people want or need from a doctor? How did they want to be served? What needs weren't being met by the conventional model?

Above all else, people wanted to spend time with their doctor. Most said they wished they had a physician who really knew them—who they were, their situation, and their health goals. Some people expressed that they wanted doctors to be available in the evenings. Some wanted to be taught how to avoid the doctor's office altogether or to wean off their medication. Dr. Wible asked if they would be willing to pay for a practice like that, and people said yes. That's the genius of this model: You pre-sell your future patients.

The way to move past fears of failure is to reach out to the community. Instead of querying fellow doctors who adhere to the dogma of the old model, physicians looking to move into functional medicine can connect with a new community. Patient-centered, relationship-driven medicine is in high demand, and members of the community are often really encouraging doctors to take the leap of faith.

There is no lack of sick people, and the number of those with chronic illness is growing each day. As more primary care practices become part of hospital systems, individual doctors have less time to spend with patients. As the system fails them, patients are driven to Functional Medicine. The challenge isn't finding patients but developing and training doctors to meet the demand.

In the old model, "build it and they will come," doctors would have to quit their job and build a physical practice before they had any idea whether it will be a success, playing directly into their financial fears. Dr. Wible's model is taught in medical schools and was featured in a Harvard School of Public Health textbook, *Renegotiating Health Care,* which examines major trends that hold the potential to change the dynamics of healthcare.

This isn't a new strategy. Various entrepreneurs, some of the most successful on the planet, would credit listening as a major part of their success. In 2016, I had the opportunity to connect with Sir Richard Branson on Necker Island, his private island in the British Virgin Islands. Thirty-four entrepreneurs, investors, and innovators were invited to learn, connect, and inspire one another to create more robust and meaningful change on the planet. The week was evidence of the importance of community to create health, and I walked away with a renewed understanding of the importance of relationships. The best advice Sir Richard gives to all entrepreneurs is to listen—to your customers and employees. Functional medicine in clinical practice is very much focused on listening, and the business model should reflect this priority.

The Lean Start Up model is often used by businesses in Silicon Valley. With this new framework, doctors can query their patients before they quit their day jobs and find out how to build a practice that their patients will want to patronize. There are many ways that you could garner feedback from your current patient base, but taking the time Dr. Wible did, providing a community forum for discussion, really made the patients feel like their opinion mattered. Similarly, you will hear in later chapters how people learn better in community. Since some people are introverts and some are extroverts who will ask the questions others are afraid to, and everyone can learn from each other.

This is the perfect start for a low overhead micropractice.

For medicine, this is a whole new way of doing business: building a community, serving the community based on what they want (as opposed to what others think they need), and creating something that people are willing to pay for. Physicians can determine whether or not it would be a viable practice before they've started building it, and patients can feel like they have been seen and heard. Similarly, there are some community members who will prove to be excellent partners down the line, such as owners of local health-related businesses like synergistic healthcare providers, health food store owners, or CrossFit trainers. Inviting those sort of people to the discussion would be a definite best practice. In fact, this type of surveying is what Seth Godin calls a "remarkable" experience, the key word being remarkable: so good you remark on it to others. Welcome to the start of your word-of-mouth practice.

We are currently at the intersection of community and medicine, and Functional Medicine is superbly positioned to be a leader in this convergence. In his book *The Daniel Plan,* Dr.

Mark Hyman shared this incredible story of his work at the Saddleback Church, and it serves as the perfect example of the awesome power that communities have when combined with functional medicine. The congregation of 15,000 already met once a week for church services, and thousands of smaller groups met again on Wednesdays for a Bible study. Infusing functional medicine ideas into this pre-existing community framework with the help of their pastor, Rick Warren, the church's population of 15,000 was able to lose a combined 250,000 pounds, and reverse various chronic diseases in the process. If functional medicine is going to be an economically viable path for health creation, then physicians and providers need to take full advantage of the power of community, especially those that are already in existence.

The existing Blue Zones Dan Buettner studied in his book do not boast numerous or expansive medical facilities. Instead, they have communities where health and well-being are a priority, and creating health is both an end goal and a daily practice. Residents often have close ties to one another— familial or otherwise—and look out for the best interests of their neighbors and the community. This social issue then translates to civic policy, with leaders responding to the needs of the people and considering their health and well-being when it comes to legislation that impacts the society and environment.

Community innovation is also emerging in reducing healthcare costs. In the current insurance model, everyone is incentivized to get as much care as they can because they're cost blind. Liberty Direct was started as an innovative way to address rising costs. At its most elemental, a group of people came together and said, "We're healthy, we want to stay healthy, and we are committing to sharing our health cost expenses within our community." If one person got hit by a car and it costs $35,000, and 35,000 of our healthy friend split costs, we would all chip in a dollar. This structure incentivizes everyone in the group to reduce their own costs and is a model worth considering as we look to create an optimal system. Although it's an innovation in healthcare and in the early phases, it has the potential to solve big-incentive problems that are currently unsolved—again, thanks to this intersection of community and medicine.

From the macro to the micro, the importance of community is reiterated in the research led by Dr. George Slavich of the UCLA Stress Lab. Through the emerging science of Human Social Genomics, only possible with the dramatic decrease in the cost of genomic sequencing, doctors and researchers have determined that the implications of social involvement or lack thereof can be seen in the expression of one's genes. Their initial research has shown that having healthy relationships—and not feeling isolated or alone—is a better predictor of good health outcomes than not smoking, proper nutrition, or regular exercise.

There is also the example of targeted rejection. If you're targeted for rejection by a social group, like being fired from your job, your chance of having depression goes up twenty times.

In comparison, a general rejection—where the whole team is fired—only sees it rise by two times. Isolation and targeted rejection significantly increases inflammatory markers and their related illnesses—from depression to heart disease, and everything in between.

Take all of that in for a moment. Social relationships are a bigger predictor of all causes of mortality than anything— even smoking, nutrition, or exercise. That is huge. In a later chapter, we'll discover how physicians can use that principle to help create communities that offer peer-to-peer support, as well as how patients can share their own wisdom, support, and resources to others looking to create health.

We have tried to model this new paradigm in our business. The Functional Forum, our monthly show, was started with the intention of connecting physicians who were interested in learning about functional medicine to those who were already practicing, and to bring down the barriers to doctors finding out about functional medicine. Wanting to foster a sense of community, the online show featured specialists and practitioners who had wisdom to share. We also wanted to bring together the communities of functional medicine and technology entrepreneurs, recognizing that functional medicine needs technology to scale up and become more efficient if it is to take its rightful place at the front lines of medicine.

The online show reduced the barrier of entry for curious practitioners around the world, where people could learn more about functional medicine without having to pay conference registration fees, take time off from work, or book flights and hotels. They could watch interviews, seminars, and even the Evolution of Medicine summit at any time on the YouTube channel, and connect with like-minded individuals online. This is a perfect example of how technology is an integral part of scaling and reproducing the model of functional medicine, and how it can allow us to create communities of doctors online before they make the switch in their own communities.

The Functional Forum is now the world's largest integrative medicine conference. Initially, we started a meet-up in New York City to get these individuals all in one room. When the Forum was livestreamed, people from all over the world were able to digitally connect. We now have over 200 meet-ups of doctors going on around the world each month, and anyone can visit meetup.functionalforum.com to learn how to start their own local group.

One of the best ways to push past the fear that practicing functional medicine is "weird" is by talking to people who have made the switch or are in the process of it. There's a wide range of medical conferences, and one could choose to attend a gastroenterology conference that brushes aside the mere mention of functional medicine, or they could choose to attend something like the Functional Forum, where people are looking to support each other in overcoming fears and creating health for themselves and their patients.

The Functional Forum allows physicians to meet people who are doing this on a regular basis and hear about their experiences, challenges, and results. Doctors who were once on the cutting edge are now ambassadors, helping others get involved. There's a lot to be learned from their trials, errors, and successes. During seminars and lectures, physicians who are new to functional medicine can receive content and resources, and follow up with group discussions. Learning is easier in community, and discussing a seminar or conference with others is valuable because everyone has a different take away from the talk. This helps everyone learn more quickly and fosters a sense of connection.

The community that is built between physicians at these meet-ups translates into the communities where they live and work. The community can be a resource in the same way the network of doctors within functional medicine can be a resource.

This in itself is remarkable, because for decades doctors and patients have been working in isolation. Doctors are often separated by modalities, siloed from those outside their fields. Medicine was founded on principles of privacy, keeping patients and doctors from seeing much of each other, and even patients were quarantined (literally or metaphorically) or not encouraged to speak to one another. Whether we look at the micro level at Dr. George Slavich's research with the UCLA Stress Lab or at the macro level with the Blue Zones, we can see that community is an important part of health and that, just like nutrition, exercise, and stress management, it is as important for doctors to model the behavior as to proselytize about it.

The forum also reiterates the importance of community—people cooking together, sharing meals, exercising in public spaces, praying together, and supporting one another in times of need—proving that a lot of health creation starts with families and small communities simply being together. The modern community micropractice provides spaces for doctors and patients to connect, and opportunities for patients to connect as well.

After the success of the Functional Forum, we used Dr. Wible's model to establish the Evolution of Medicine Practice Accelerator. We asked doctors of functional medicine what they wanted to learn about managing and growing their practices, as well as what challenges they faced and what frustrated them. They responded by saying they wanted to know how to create better patient education systems, how to use more efficient procedures, how to increase revenue, and how to create a consistent flow of incoming patients.

Once we knew what the issues were, we could create a program that specifically addressed them. Physicians were a priceless resource to help us determine how best to provide value to them and their practice, and the process allowed them to trust us more. Without their input, we wouldn't have created something that met their needs. To do so, we had to ask questions and listen very carefully to the answers. Functional medicine needs to work in that way—speaking to the patients, finding out what their needs are, and then building a practice or a treatment plan around that.

This can be done online or it can be done in person. Either way, it doesn't need a lot of bells and whistles—not even an office. There's no reason not to start taking steps toward the goal when the resources are free and easily accessible. No one needs to attend a conference or quit their day job to start learning or talking to patients. All it takes is time and interest, and what that looks like varies for everyone. Start by talking to patients, or by watching YouTube videos and checking out the resources recommended by speakers—Mark Hyman's books, for instance. Eventually, it's helpful to connect with other physicians online, having back-and-forth discussions about functional medicine, which could lead to attending a conference or training program. There's no right or wrong way to go about learning or integrating functional medicine into a physician's practice. In the same way that functional medicine treats the individual, the resources that are available cater to various learning styles and levels. When someone is ready to learn more, functional medicine provides structured and systematic training and education, making the model both scalable and repeatable.

Even though we created the Functional Forum to be watched anywhere, doctors still like to attend a range of conferences on functional medicine, because it allows people to connect with their tribe. In the next chapter, we're going to share some of the options to receive training to feel more a part of this emerging community.

QUESTION: *What is my community looking for in a practice?*

ACTION: *Find a way to gather feedback from the community.*

CHAPTER FOUR

TRAINING AND EDUCATION

*"Holism is the tendency in nature to form wholes greater
than the sum of the parts through creative evolution."*
——JAN SMUTS, Prime Minister of South Africa

I N 2005 DR. ROBYNNE Chutkan developed the flu just before
going into labor with her first child. After sixteen hours and
a high fever, doctors tried labor-inducing drugs to no avail
and finally performed a C-section. Doctors then decided that
Dr. Chutkan's newborn should be placed in the neonatal ICU
(NICU) as a precautionary measure. Though the baby was
perfectly healthy, doctors gave her two strong intravenous
antibiotics just in case. At the time, Dr. Chutkan thought it
was great to see them being so proactive.

At about six months old, the baby started developing infections, had her first episode of a fever and sore throat, and was diagnosed with pharyngitis. This was her first course of what would be "many, many, many courses of antibiotics"—about fifteen courses in the next two and a half years. She was hospitalized for rotavirus, treated for non-draining fluid in her ear, and had prolonged coughs during the winter months. After one visit, her daughter was prescribed an antibiotic, a steroid, an antihistamine, a bronchodilator, and given a nebulizer machine. They had visited the doctor fifty times before she even entered kindergarten. Dr. Chutkan knew they needed a different approach, and like Dr. Gladd, she was convinced that there had to be a better way.

Dr. Robynne Chutkan was trained as a gastroenterologist two decades ago. When she graduated in 1991, germs were still considered "our foes," rather than "a really integral part of our body's ecology." Though the microbiome is mainly housed in the gut, the organ she specialized in, no one was talking about it, and Dr. Chutkan said, "The term didn't even exist when I was in medical school." Fifteen years ago, people would say they had inflammatory bowel disease because of the antibiotics and non-steroidals they were taking, and Dr. Chutkan and her colleagues thought it was nonsense. Fast-forward to 2014, when Mount Sinai Hospital in New York released a study that stated frequent usage of antibiotics like Cipro was "strongly associated with new onset of Crohn's disease." Dr. Chutkan pointed out, "The irony here is that these are two antibiotics we frequently use to treat these conditions."

It wasn't just the antibiotics that concerned Dr. Chutkan. "C-sections bypass this really critical early step in the maturation of the microbiome," she says. Though it wasn't evident then, when we now "look at the microbiome of babies born via C-section, we find that they're colonized with hospital-associated bacteria like staph versus the vaginally born babies who tend to be colonized with lactobacillus and other more beneficial species." Dr. Chutkan now realizes that "how [we] enter the world really has profound implications later on."

Her child first helped open her eyes, and her patients fomented her desire to know more about what was going on. She notes that because doctors are taught in conventional and traditional models, they can be slow to adopt new ideas. She recommends that doctors "keep an open mind and listen" to patients, even if they "say things that sound outlandish and far-fetched, because a few years later, you'll often find out that they're correct. [...] We're moving at a thousand miles an hour in terms of what we're finding out."

Even though science is evolving quicker than ever before, it still takes seventeen years for new science to be adopted into mainstream medicine. We are quickly making new connections, such as the relationship between microbes, antibiotics, and chronic inflammation. For instance, research is being done on the "gut-brain axis" or how the gut and the brain impact one another, and we're now seeing that the two are intrinsically connected through the vagus nerve. Doctors of functional medicine are creating structures whereby one can understand the body as an integrated system, and then go upstream to determine the least possible intervention that begets the maximum possible impact on these systems, which appeals to both accountants and those who value elegant solutions.

Once you start looking through the systems thinking approach, you see the connections everywhere. If chronic diseases are multi-systemic, then systems thinking becomes paramount. Until we have a "supergeneralist" residency in every medical school in the world, functional medicine is the quickest way to train this increasingly necessary wing of the medical system.

This is the *Evolution of Medicine*, medicine adapting to its new environment through the path of least resistance. There is a unique opportunity at this juncture in history to train physician-entrepreneurs to establish practices grounded in functional medicine before the biggest medical stakeholders catch on. In what other industry, at what other time, was there a greater opportunity for entrepreneurs to practice today's medicine and build a successful business in this new paradigm?

Later in the book, we will get into the best practices for running the low overhead "Functional Micropractice" off a laptop, but first and foremost, there is a need for some clinical education. Over two online summits and 30 episodes of our live show, we have showcased many of the core ideas, but our intention with our content was only to light a spark underneath practitioners and guide them to the best training programs for them.

In fact, there are so many options for training that it can be daunting for doctors looking for a way in that suits them. At the Evolution of Medicine, we have attempted to be a "consumer reports" style service for clinicians and other health professionals who want to join the Functional Medicine movement to find the right resources to accelerate that shift for them. Those resources typically fit into three categories: clinical education, practice management training programs, and best in category technologies. I mean, do you really have time to sit through 50 electronic medical record (EMR) demos to know the right questions to ask?

At the end of this chapter is a link to a special video we have created that goes over the various functional medicine trainings, their duration, pricing, key benefits, and drawbacks. Within all of these trainings, doctors learn about systems biology—the concept that the body is a web, as opposed to separate organs operating in isolation. Instead of separating the organs, functional medicine considers their interdependence and relationships. Each of the trainings will vary in delivery and format, but all five of those mentioned below get consistently great feedback from their students.

There are a number of education choices in functional medicine, and in fact we have seen more and more well curated conferences popping up all over the world over the last five years. This is by no means an exhaustive list, and if you have a special interest in environmental medicine, mind-body medicine, genomics, methylation, or the microbiome, there are niche conferences that might be a perfect start.

1. THE INSTITUTE FOR FUNCTIONAL MEDICINE (IFM) was founded by Dr. Jeffrey Bland and Susan Bland in 1991 and established a lot of elements that are a big part of functional medicine education today, such as the Functional Medicine timeline and matrix. Dr. Leo Galland developed the patient-centered diagnosis, and Dr. Bob Rountree, among others, was integral to the creation of the matrix. One of the core strengths of the IFM is that it draws on the know-how of a community of pioneering doctors, too many to name here. Their introductory course, "Applying Functional Medicine in a Clinical Practice," is a comprehensive overview of the Functional Medicine Matrix, and the systems biology approach to understanding and treating chronic disease. That's meant to be a foundational course, and there are other modules that allow practitioners to deepen their knowledge over time, including focuses on immunity, hormone imbalances, gastrointestinal equilibrium, toxicity, metabolic and cardiovascular issues, and pain management. Additionally, IFM organizes an international conference, runs a certification program, and recently expanded to offer e-learning courses for practitioners who can't travel to study.

2. FUNCTIONAL MEDICINE UNIVERSITY (FMU) offers online continuing education for physicians that are meant to be completed at one's chosen pace. Courses cater to various styles of learning, so those who are auditory learners can listen to recordings, while visual learners can enjoy slides, handouts, or videos. Functional Medicine University has been particularly popular among Chiropractors in the US and Canada, as well as international doctors of all disciplines, since the content is all online and requires no travel. FMU puts out plenty of free clinical content to give you a flavor of their training.

3. THE KRESSER INSTITUTE was launched by Chris Kresser in 2015 to help doctors replicate his successful practice in Berkeley, California. The course is one year long and combines functional medicine with an evolutionary approach to health, as well as insight into his clinic's micropractice structure, digital toolbox, and case studies. Chris Kresser's trainings focus on both the clinical and organizational sides of the practice, and are a combination of online resources and four in-person trainings over the year.

4. HOLISTIC NUTRITION LAB focuses on trainings and resources for nutritionists, acupuncturists, health coaches, and nurses—all reaches of the healthcare industry. These kinds of providers can't order labs, so that restriction has led to a new discipline of functional nutrition. The same kinds of structures that work in functional medicine—the timeline and the matrix—are used here, and this is a

great way to get the rest of your provider team to speak a common language. One remarkable thing Holistic Nutrition Lab has created is the online community, where practitioners solve each other's problems, and founder Andrea Nakayama provides a ton of regular contribution.

5. DR. DAN KALISH has been providing mentorship and systems for doctors to thrive in functional medicine for over a decade. In 2016, a group of Mayo Clinic researchers validated his system for dealing with the common ailments in functional medicine practice. Dr. Kalish's program is very heavy on the development of practice systems and has helped many providers build sustainable practices quickly.

Make sure to check out the video listing at the end of this chapter that gives the prices, timings, travel options, and durations for these different organizations. Whichever of these trainings you chose, you will find all sorts of useful tools, resources, and clinical tips to help patients cover the most basic areas of health creation: exercise, stress reduction, healthy sleep, and anti-inflammatory diets. Beyond that, the trainings venture into how to prioritize interventions for the individual and the quickest ways to build function in different organs and systems through therapeutic supplementation.

"We need the medicine of etiology, not symptomatology" said Dr. Rangan Chatterjee at the end of his TEDx talk. "If we only treat symptoms, we'll never get rid of the disease." At the core of common chronic diseases are the same root causes.

Diet, stress levels, chronic sleep deprivation, physical inactivity, lack of sun exposure, and disruption of the gut and microbiome—all of these are underlying factors for almost all chronic inflammatory diseases like type 2 diabetes, depression, and even dementia.

Another massive feature of functional medicine is *root cause resolution*. I had never heard that term until Dr. Kelly Brogan and I went onto HuffPost Live to promote the Evolution of Medicine Summit in 2014. That led to a whole Functional Forum on the topic in April 2015. This term seems to resonate with family physicians and specialists alike, who tend to have a nagging feeling they aren't able to help patients truly overcome their condition. When the acute care framework is applied to chronic diseases of lifestyle origin, neither the patient, provider, or payer end up happy. (Except the US, since the Affordable Care Act [ACA] introduced the 80/20 rule of health insurance and a system of perverse incentives went into hyperdrive!)

But what are these root causes? The story of Dr. Chutkan's daughter is a perfect example of how something at birth or in childhood can lead to other health issues down the line. Most doctors wouldn't connect antibiotics given at birth to symptoms that occur twenty years later. C-section babies, as Dr. Chutkan pointed out, miss out on microbes within the birth canal that are vitally important later in life. Similarly, Dr. Chutkan notes that babies raised on formula aren't provided human milk oligosaccharides (HMOs) that are present in breast milk. Although babies can't digest HMOs, they are a growth medium for the baby's bacteria, bifidobacteria infantis, which nourishes the baby's microbiome.

In what current medical system would that be connected to a gastrointestinal issue or a mental health issue or a rheumatological issue? Never. But the newest science is showing you can affect gut, brain, and joints through interventions based on improving gut ecology. Only functional medicine, with its comprehensive timeline and lengthy intake form, is able not only to make the connection, but also to provide the support needed to fix the cause of the problem.

"This is preventative medicine in its purest form. We have got to stop applying twentieth century thinking to twenty-first century problems." Dr. Chatterjee summarized this perfectly at the end of his talk.

It is certainly preventative medicine, but any medical system built on systems biology must also be holistic, even though that word has been bastardized since its original use. Former South African Prime Minister Jan Smuts coined the word *holism* in 1935: "The tendency in nature to form wholes greater than the sum of the parts *through creative evolution*." What could be a more perfect example of creative evolution than that of our relationship with our gut bacteria? We need them, and they need us, and the sooner we all start acting like it, the better.

QUESTION: *How well-equipped is your practice to consistently create health?*

ACTION: *Go to goevomed.com/functional to watch a five-minute video about different options for functional medicine training.*

CHAPTER FIVE

TEST AND CHALLENGES

*"It's supposed to be difficult, it's a shortcut! If it were
easy it would just be the way."*

— *ROAD TRIP* movie

D R. JEFFREY GLADD STARTED incorporating functional
medicine into his practice slowly, by spending more time
with patients and asking them about their nutrition, sleep
patterns, work, and relationships. He found that 80% weren't
very interested and mainly wanted their prescription and to
go home. The other 20% were really interested in furthering
discussions of health creation, but the way Dr. Gladd's practice
was structured couldn't always accommodate that.

After training with Dr. Andrew Weil at the University of Arizona's Center for Integrative Medicine, Dr. Gladd asked his local hospital if they could start an integrative medicine program. Surprisingly and graciously, they accepted, and Dr. Gladd worked with them to get it off the ground. They were very successful when it came to patient satisfaction and engagement, and had a six-month waiting list of people trying to get in. Dr. Gladd was healthier than ever, and much happier and more fulfilled in his work.

However, billing insurance for sixty- to ninety-minute office visits proved challenging. "Financially it wasn't a success at all," Dr. Gladd said. Ultimately, the hospital said that although they loved what he did, he would need to see three times more patients in order for it to continue. Since that wasn't feasible within the model they had constructed, the program was shut down, and Dr. Gladd went on to start his own practice.

The University of Arizona's Center for Integrative Medicine opened an integrative primary care clinic in 2012 with District Medical Group as an operating partner—the university can't directly operate clinics, according to state law. The clinic was meant to be a pilot program to observe challenges, benefits, and costs. The demand was more than they could accommodate, and the clinic served 1,800 patients, with 700 enrolling in an outcomes study, which showed the practice's significant impacts on the health of the community.

Despite these successes, Dr. Victoria Maizes and Dr. Andrew

Weil announced in 2016 that the clinic would close at the end of July. The university's operating partner decided to "focus on other opportunities" and another potential operating partner had "too many competing priorities" to take over the innovative clinic.

Responding to the closure in an e-mail, Dr. Jeffrey Gladd said it was "yet another reason why progressive models of care have to be embraced." Meaning that practitioners need to think outside the box when it comes to the structure of their integrative clinics. "I'm not sure integrative care models can be large scale, or bill insurance to be successful," Dr. Gladd wrote. "We need lots of small, artisanal, creative practices."

Back in 2014, Dr. Gladd mentioned in an interview that doctors interested in learning more about functional medicine often approach him to ask his opinions on trainings or certifications. His advice comes with a disclaimer: "I caution them, and let them know that—at some level—the knowledge is fantastic for your personal health. But it could be a curse for your professional health and for your career."

For Dr. Gladd, practicing functional medicine inside a conventional model—especially one that dealt with insurance—was frustrating. The excitement and idealism post-training can be challenged by the realities of finances—having to decide between an insurance model or a cash-pay model, for instance, or needing to hire administrative staff to handle billing and insurance. According to *Healthline*, "In 2013, a *Harvard Business*

Review analysis showed the healthcare workforce has grown by 75% since 1990, but 95% of new hires aren't doctors. The ratio of doctors to other healthcare workers is now 1:16, up from 1:14 two decades ago. Of those sixteen workers for every doctor, only six are involved for caring for patients—nurses and home health aides, for example. The other ten are purely administrative roles."

Many doctors go through training programs and quickly realize they don't work in a business model that allows them to implement it into functional medicine. In some cases, an employer won't let them do it because it's not as financially viable as their model, and doctors who run their own practices also find it hard to scale up efficiently and increase revenue with themselves as typically the only "producer." Although patients and practitioners alike love functional medicine, the business structure of the old model doesn't allow people to dive into it.

In May 2016, the Institute for Functional Medicine released the results of the first-ever large-scale practice survey where physicians were asked about nonclinical aspects of their practice. The results were staggering. The last five years have seen a massive uptick in interest in functional medicine. The survey also showed higher rates of satisfaction for doctors, with many wanting to continue practicing well past retirement and into their seventies.

However, this was counterbalanced with the statistics that some functional medicine doctors weren't earning as much as their primary care or family medicine colleagues, never mind the massive wealth of top specialists. Many were struggling to create a successful practice model, and there were big disparities in income, especially around two key factors. Doctors who saw themselves as early technology adopters earned an average of $50,000 per year more than those who took the opposite view, and it was another $50,000 for those who felt comfortable charging patients for services earned vs. those who didn't.

This can affirm a lot of physicians' worst fears. As mentioned in Chapter 2, a lot of doctors are afraid of failing financially. Getting a practice up off the ground only to see it crash and burn can be devastating. There have been a lot of practice wreckage and many failed practices in the first era of functional medicine, and it has been a burden on the pace of the movement. When you start to practice with a fundamentally different type of care, you need a new model for delivering it. This took a lot of trial and error from a lot of people, but as I said before, we've seen enough practices start and run successfully to know that it can be done—and with the effective use of technology it can be reproduced and scaled much more easily.

According to the survey 75% of functional medicine doctors had cash-pay practices, realizing that the insurance model was tricky to implement sustainably when practicing functional medicine, with only 20% operating within the insurance system and 5% using one of the new direct primary care (DPC) style membership models. There are great individual examples of practices of how each model thrives, and we have featured many on our podcasts. We are only just starting to see emerging best practices, and what I have coined "Functional Medicine 2.0," though most of the credit for that term goes to Dr. Gladd.

My good friend Tom Blue, the chief strategy officer of the American Academy of Private Physicians and a key supporter of the Evolution of Medicine, points out that health creation delivered by functional medicine is not expensive, especially when compared to costs of prescription drugs, surgeries, and the long-term treatment of symptoms. Never mind the cost to the insurer—sometimes just the copays for drugs can be hundreds of dollars a month. Humira, anyone? Patients and physicians are often cost-blind when it comes to services, because everything is coded to insurance, passed back and forth between a physician and the insurance, and shrouded in secrecy. With insurance premiums rising out of control, how long will it be until patients and companies (for whom medical costs are typically the second largest cost after payroll) just run out of money?

The economics of functional medicine make a lot more sense for chronic disease, and the most progressive thinkers in medicine see a future split between chronic and acute disease. Hospitals are designed for acute disease, and they do a phenomenal job in that realm. But the economics of chronic disease will bankrupt us all unless we go upstream and deliver truly participatory medicine.

There are examples of successful functional medicine clinics taking insurance, but they are few and far between. I have heard such horror stories of time wasted on the phone and fax machines and doctors either waiting months to get paid or in some cases, having money taken directly from bank accounts when the payer made changes in their payment terms with little or no notice. This is not an environment in which entrepreneurs thrive.

One of the most successful examples is Dr. Ornish's "Intensive Cardiac Rehab" program, which pays for over 100 hours of care, split over six providers and paying over $7,000 per patient for nine weeks of care. And that's on Medicare—commercial insurers will often pay slightly more. To pull off this program you have to have not only the team capable of delivering it, but also a big enough list of cardiac patients to make it work for everyone, so large cardiology groups could easily add this to their menu of services.

One option outside the realm of insurance is the cash-pay model. Dr. Jeffrey Gladd incorporated this into his own practice. "I decided that I didn't want to work for the healthcare system, or the hospital, or even the insurance companies. I wanted to work for patients."

His practice is set up in Fort Wayne, Indiana, which *Men's Health* once rated the dumbest city in the country. *USA Today* titled an article about the town, "Looking for signs of intelligent life in Fort Wayne." In the middle of a recession in the so-called dumbest city in the country, Dr. Gladd created a successful community-focused cash model practice. He spends as much time with a patient as they need, focusing on the patient's goals and priorities. He's been doing this for six years now with great success, seeing twenty-five to thirty new patients each month, and working no more than three days per week in the clinic. He equates it to a lemonade stand—doctors have something of value, and patients are happy to pay for it.

This was echoed by Dr. Lorraine Page, who said, "It's just lovely. The patients do better, I get to see the whole person, the whole family. It's true family practice. And it's very straightforward. I see the person, I get paid. It's simple."

The healthcare system blinds doctors and patients to the cost of services. Doctors are told that the hospitals, administration, and insurance will take care of it so they can simply focus on practicing medicine. Dr. Gladd discussed this at a Functional Forum talk in 2014, where he told the story of a patient who had initially gone to a cardiologist. The patient spent no more than ten minutes with the cardiologist, who said his cholesterol levels were normal. The patient had a $2,200 out-of-pocket invoice from the hospital for those ten minutes, which went toward meeting his deductible. With more and more people on high-deductible plans, this is more common than you'd imagine.

In contrast, Dr. Gladd sat down with the same patient to discuss options and costs—how much labs would be with and without insurance, as well as specialized tests and services.

Dr. Gladd ran a full NMR lipid profile, homocysteine, and high-sensitivity C-reactive protein, and spent a full hour reviewing what the results meant with the patient. They discussed what shifts in lifestyle he could make to help improve the numbers. After all was said and done, it cost a fourth of what he paid for ten minutes with the cardiologist.

Recent data showed the average Functional Medicine patient has six diagnoses and thirty symptoms, which makes them a pretty interesting niche in medicine. Treating all of these symptoms separately, with separate specialists, would take a lot of time and money. Functional medicine can assist those who need it most by providing "supergeneralists" and care aimed at improving function, not symptom whack-a-mole. Dr. Gladd's example between his practice and the cardiologist's illustrates this perfectly.

A cash-pay practice means doctors need to learn skills they weren't taught in medical school. With the insurance system, doctors never have to deal with money. With a cash practice, physicians need to become comfortable discussing costs openly and honestly, as well as charging patients and performing transactions. It's definitely a behavioral shift, but that doesn't mean it needs to happen overnight. This is another reason why slowly transitioning to a functional medicine practice—starting one day a week and scaling up—is a great idea.

A slightly different approach to fee-for-service is the package model, which works for patients with chronic conditions. If a patient has type 2 diabetes that they want to get under control, progressive functional medicine clinics can set up a package where, for a certain amount, they'll receive a set number of services for a predetermined amount of time. That could be one-on-one appointments with the doctor, labs and supplements, group classes for support, time with a nutritionist and diabetes specialist, and an educational curriculum. Think of it as a customizable course for chronic disease, where patients educate themselves on how to create health. This is participatory medicine at its finest, and when patients pay in advance, they are often more committed to the course of action. Innovative clinics are providing financing options to make these packages more affordable.

Another option outside of insurance is direct primary care (DPC) or membership models, and this is a conversation that we at the Evolution of Medicine are thrilled to be in the center of. Fee-for-service was designed for acute care, and although some doctors like Dr. Gladd have been able to pull it off successfully, it is clear that financial relationships that match how the care is received make a lot of sense.

Direct primary care is often confused with concierge medicine, which tends to be more expensive. With direct primary care, doctors never bill insurance, whereas concierge medicine bills insurance, and patients pay a monthly retainer for noncovered services, ranging from $2,000 to $30,000 a year. Direct primary care charges a relatively small monthly fee.

A recent article pointed out that "the lack of overhead in direct primary care allows doctors to keep a greater share of the money coming in, even if they make less overall than in a traditional practice." Dr. Wible said, "My expenses are so low, they're now about 10 percent of my practice, [...] And it used to be 74 percent."

Dr. Lorraine Page echoed this: "At our office, we had six full-time doctors. And we had seven full-time insurance people, [...] So [that's] more than one full-time person trying to get reimbursement for patients I was seeing." She now provides direct primary care, doesn't take insurance, and mostly operates in cash.

Dr. Robin Berzin's Parsley Health that started in New York is the perfect example of this model. Dr. Berzin charges patients $150 a month to have access to ongoing care throughout the year and unlimited access to her team of health coaches. If a patient falls ill and needs to visit a few times in a month, the fee is still $150. If a patient feels well and doesn't come it at all, the fee is still $150 per month. I'm sure you've heard the story of Chinese doctors who only got paid when people were well, and not when they got sick. This seems to me to be the closest model I've seen to that structure, which seems intuitive and resonates with both patients and providers alike.

Parsley Health's monthly fee incentivizes people to visit as much or as little as they feel comfortable. Either way, the rate is consistent. This aligns well with her policy that patients can't make just one appointment. She writes about this in articles and blogs, reiterating that one appointment won't help someone looking to reverse a chronic ailment or practice true prevention. As my good friend Dr. Datis Kharrazian says, "Don't build a car repair shop if you are trying to build a driving school." In a patient's first appointment, Dr. Berzin will spend a lot of time on the intake form with the patient, but without a follow up, all that information is pretty much useless. The inherent value of functional medicine is having a different kind of doctor-patient relationship, in which patients are empowered, educated, committed to the process, and participatory.

When patients pay doctors by the hour, it can de-incentivize health creation, in the same way that high deductibles and expensive co-pays keep people from visiting more than once per year. Although functional medicine practitioners sometimes use hourly models, people with chronic illnesses may be less inclined to come in if they're paying by the hour.

As Chief Strategy Officer of the American Academy of Private Physicians, Tom Blue has been at the cutting edge of this topic for more than a decade. Some of his most important observations of chronic care concern the fact that patients respond to their environment—if they're on the clock whenever they see a provider, they want to minimize that. He likens it to meeting with lawyers—the person paying the bill doesn't want to spend any more time than they have to when they're on the clock. DPC can help patients get off the clock, put the money on the back burner of the relationship, and create a more authentic connection that responds to people's needs without hurting their wallets.

Another friend of mine, Dr. Heba Elnazer, a young doctor in Cairo, built an integrated medicine center after training in the United States. After a few iterations of the business model, she pivoted to a direct primary care and membership practice. Patients flocked to her, and investors asked how they could help scale it across the country. The membership model—where people pay a certain amount per month and have access when they need it—is working as a new way to deliver care all over the world. Evolutionarily, we all know how meaningful it is to be a member of a tribe, and the best DPC practices look to conjure that atmosphere with member events and group experiences.

For doctors, this model means consistent income. Four hundred members who pay $150 per month will earn the clinic a steady $60,000 in monthly revenue and are likely to be able to be serviced by one doctor. That predictable income means knowing you can cover any overhead costs each month, and know how many members are in the practice at any given time. Traditional practices may have over 2,000 patients on the books, but they couldn't say how many are still living in the area or will want to book an appointment on a certain day, week, or month. It's unclear who they are responsible for, whereas in the membership model, doctors know who is counting on them.

Over the years, I've met many doctors whose retirement plan is to sell their practice to a new doctor. The problem is, the value of a practice is anticipated future revenue streams, and when one doctor's practice passes to another, there can be few guarantees of patients continuing to visit. Within a membership structure, it's easier to predict future revenue streams, and the value of a practice skyrockets. For all of these reasons, we feel that functional medicine and direct primary care are a great match.

One concern with direct primary care and fees is that the approach excludes low-income patients, especially those who count on Medicare or Medicaid for coverage. The models of functional medicine are evolving to meet these needs, and can be flexible. I've seen $60 a month models in the deep South that are frequented by low-income families, and I've seen $250 a month clinics in Connecticut, and each can work financially, depending on the service mix of each membership tier. In our recent two-day course, "Building Your Functional Medicine Membership Practice" (which will soon be available online), Tom Blue gave practitioners all the tools to model this transition to membership, including budgeting for time, overhead, and salary.

Superimposing functional medicine with the conventional operating system leads to a lot of problems and challenges— such as being able to see enough patients and maintain a financially viable, sustainable practice. Addressing these challenges means thinking outside the box and considering alternative methods and practices, like direct primary care.

Tom Blue says, "Direct primary care is the best business model for private medicine, and functional medicine is the best clinical model for creating health, and for the first time there's an opportunity to put the two together." Within direct primary care, if you're just spending more time with patients and putting them on the same drugs, then it isn't really an improvement in the model. Likewise, if you're practicing functional medicine in the old business model, it's de-incentivizing the right relationship.

We don't need a slow-motion version of our current medical system, because it's not empowering health or changing behaviors. Direct primary care and functional medicine together create the time and space for participatory medicine, where patients are engaged in their own care. That is what ultimately leads to awesome and powerful change.

Above all, the models that are flourishing are micropractices—low-overhead, technologically-enabled practices in a community setting. Dr. Jeffrey Gladd transitioned away from working with a large hospital to start his own practice, which had a low overhead and used technology to help it run more efficiently. He works only three days per week in the office, because doctors can now work securely and remotely with the use of new technologies. He can pick his kids up from school and take Fridays off to spend the weekend with his family.

Dr. Robin Berzin's practice at Parsley Health also started as a micropractice, which allows her to cut down on costs like owning or leasing a building. Instead, she can rent a space for a few days a week and work remotely the rest of the time. The membership fee allows for predictable income and a strong foundation for her bigger vision.

Dr. Alejandra Carrasco of nourishmedicine.com had to take a year off between medical school and her residency due to her own health issues. She had developed severe anxiety, migraines, and IBS during medical school and had to take a functional approach to healing herself before she could work on healing others. After hearing me speak in 2011, Dr. Carrasco started a low-overhead micropractice. Her office is now in an 80-square-foot space in Casa de Luz, a school, yoga studio, and macrobiotic cafe in Austin, Texas. She has fallen back in love with medicine, and her practice enables her to have time and energy for her two children. A micropractice is a great way to ensure a proper work-life balance.

Dr. Gladd tells all his patients, "I'm trying to put myself out of business. I know there's enough patients to not have that happen in my lifetime, but for you, as a patient of mine, I don't want you to see me long-term." Instead, he aims to give patients "the tools and resources" to help them "achieve a level of health" that they want. Dr. Gladd hits the mark with his approach, but I think there is a slightly different point that is sometimes missed. If the ultimate goal of functional medicine is to create healthy people who don't need constant care, then a membership model seems to be the most elegant solution for the payer and patient, because both patient and provider are incentivized to create health. If patients recover their health through the initial help of a doctor, they will stay with the practice because of the huge value it provided, while the doctor is capturing the value offered without providing more services.

Ultimately, we need to think outside the fee-for-service box to empower patients to create health by giving them the tools and resources they need. "Patient engagement is the next blockbuster drug" says Michael Dermer, an incentive expert on the Functional Forum. If this is the case we need to pull out all the stops to acquire such engagement, and that might require a business model more suited to this paradigm. In the end, participatory medicine is what will help us eradicate chronic diseases and create Blue Zones.

QUESTION: *What does financial security look like? What is your retirement plan?*

ACTION: *Schedule time to update your business plan. Or write a new one.*

CHAPTER SIX

PATIENT EDUCATION

*"The doctor of the future will give no medication, but
will interest his patients in the care of the human frame,
diet and in the cause and prevention of disease."*

— THOMAS ALVA EDISON

THE LATIN ROOT OF doctor is *docere,* to teach. Part of what
excites doctors is learning and being able to transmit
their knowledge to people to help them make the journey to
sustainable health. The current business of medicine doesn't
prioritize patient education, but functional medicine is based
on participatory care, in which patients are the heroes of their
own journeys. If we want to help patients in this way, we
have to curate relevant information that empowers people
to participate in creating health.

One of the biggest systemic inefficiencies of functional medicine up until now was that the physician was both doctor and teacher, needing to spend a lot of one-on-one time together. This is really time-consuming, not financially viable for every practice, and not always affordable for a patient. If doctors are paid by the hour, patients may be paying a lot of money to learn subjects that they could easily learn in other, more scaled, accessible ways.

Clinics and hospitals started using handouts as a way to transmit information to patients. Although this upped the scale of education, it wasn't always engaging. Handouts aren't environmentally friendly and were often badly designed or unprofessional. With the rise of technology, new avenues have arrived to efficiently educate patients, most of which are automated and take none of the doctor's time.

Let's take a moment to imagine a new reality.

Imagine you meet someone at a dinner party you get to talking about your newfound interest in functional medicine. You tell them you'll be opening a clinic, and they ask for your business card. Instead, you say, "Let me send you a quick e-mail with some information." (Yes, you might need to throw away your business cards!) Newsletter platforms like MailChimp and GetResponse have mobile apps, so you don't even need a website to start a mailing list of interested parties. You add the acquaintance's e-mail address to a mailing list on your phone and send an automated, organized, follow-up e-mail three hours later that says, "It was so great to meet you. I'll send you more information about my practice tomorrow morning. Thanks for your interest." At eight o'clock the next morning, a welcome e-mail is sent to your new acquaintance—the first of two e-mails. These are called "the perfect welcome," and in them, you craft the perfect story of your practice: why you choose to practice medicine differently, what led you to set up this practice, and links to some of your favorite resources that might help them lead healthier lives.

In the second e-mail, delivered the next day, you follow up with information about functional medicine, what to expect from a visit and all the other things you find yourself repeating a hundred times a month. The e-mail includes a well-produced video of you at your most inspiring and informative. After watching the video, your new acquaintance books an appointment through your online scheduler via a link in the second e-mail.

Congratulations, you have just delivered the next generation of patient education, and the beauty of it is that it doubles as marketing. A fully automated patient-education system that everyone goes through at the beginning of their interaction with the practice ensures that each person is introduced or on-boarded in a consistent way. Everyone will have the same resources and information sent to them, which saves a physician from having to explain the same points to each patient, and also saves the patient from having to do their own research on a doctor's website. It's a super-efficient process in which every patient receives education in bite-sized chunks. Learning one new thing a day is preferable to a dozen, especially when we consider that most will retain or remember only 5 to 10% of what was said. Instead of an hour-long appointment, clients are given the same content for five minutes a day over the course of twelve days. The beauty of videos, articles, and podcasts is that they can be listened to many times.

This is a win-win for patients and physicians. Patients receive a ton of value for free, and practitioners only need to set this up once for it to run forever. It saves time for both parties. Patients don't need to make a special trip to a doctor's office and learn new material on their own time—which is especially helpful for individuals with chronic disease who may not be able to make it to frequent appointments. All the best autoresponder sequences will curate longer resources in different mediums like articles, videos, and podcasts to make learning easy for every patient, no matter their learning style.

The autoresponder is a crucial step on the hero's journey. In the e-mail sequence, you're educating people about functional medicine and helping patients realize they are the hero of this journey—and that they need to participate in their care. You write the e-mail in a way to call them to adventure, that there might be a better way to help their condition.

Of course, it's important that clients still be able to speak with their doctor when they have questions and concerns. Some doctors are now using new technologies to connect with patients online, through HIPAA-compliant platforms to maintain confidentiality. Face-to-face time is crucial, but it doesn't always need to be with a physician. Instead, patients can work with a health coach as part of a plan outlined by their doctor. Encouraging patients to work with health coaches means physicians are free to spend time with other patients, and patients often benefit financially, as the cost of a health coach is usually much less expensive than doctor visits.

Health coaches provide support, teaching what the patient most needs to learn. That could be nutrition, exercise, meditation, or better understanding of their chronic disease or ailment. Coaches can create handouts, coordinate group visits, facilitate discussions, and run orientations. With the majority of education done by automated e-mail campaigns less time is spent in didactic teaching. This leaves the coach with more time to answer specific questions and deliver experiential learning (grocery tour anyone?).

This new system allows for more efficiency of face-to-face communications, but in different ways than the conventional model. Another option is group meet-ups, where patients with chronic diseases can meet up with other patients in either a purely educational setting or even a Medicare-sanctioned group visit. Together, patients can work toward shared and individual health goals, share wisdom, and provide support and accountability. This is something we see in Blue Zones—communities working together to create health. These same structures are being re-created in clinics across the country, although we have nowhere near seen the actualization of the potential of the group interaction to scale care. Amazing results have been seen where survivors of cancer meet with patients to discuss treatment and answer any questions, or when parents of kids with chronic health problems meet to share information.

A mother whose child has had autism for ten years can attend community meetings to share their experiences of caring for their child or family members. Other parents whose children have new diagnoses can learn from the more experienced members of the community, including how to ensure they're taking medications, how to help them eat well, what foods help or hurt behaviors, how to cope with new schools or birthday parties, and everything in between. Having been through it before, people can reflect on what they learned, what worked for them, and what they would have done differently, and this adds value to both participants, the sharer and the listener.

In groups of patients, an experienced person can share practical information with the inexperienced. Often this is more valuable and comprehensive than what a physician can cover in one hour. If a doctor hasn't been through it themselves, they can't speak to the complexities and nuances of the situation like another patient can. People who are able to teach what they've learned can feel so fulfilled, knowing they're giving back to a community that once helped them. It's ultimately much easier to heal and create health in relationship to others, freely receiving from and giving support to those who understand. Those interactions are highly valued by patients and work toward building community, which we'll come back to in Chapter 8.

The Internet is a valuable resource for patient education. Doctors can create and curate educational assets for patients, catering them to individual needs. Dr. Frank Lipman's blog is one example of free information that current and prospective patients alike often read and reread. The most effective practices take into account that everyone learns differently, and then they curate a wide range of formats—blogs, videos, podcasts, articles, and links. The beauty of videos, articles, and podcasts is that they can be listened to many times, allowing patients to retain more information.

Patient education is the first step and needs to be grounded in practice. Some patients will just need to be told what to do, others will need to be coached, and others will still need a lot of hand-holding through the process. Practices have to have resources for each individual and his or her learning style. This needs to be determined during the intake process, along with the patient's preferred learning style—auditory, visual, kinesthetic, or a mix of the three.

"How do you like to learn?" is a great question on intake forms. My friend Dr. Pedram Shojai says his "ears have more free time than [his] eyes," and prefers audio content. I'm sure there are a lot more like him. Accommodating different learning styles and varying the content increases engagement. Patients become more likely to learn and integrate it into their daily lives.

The same setup can send patients automated, organized e-mails on how to best create health. Dr. Sachin Patel of the Living Proof Institute does this with his series, "30 Ways in 30 Days." For thirty days, community members can receive encouragement and content that aligns with the mission and vision of a physician's practice. Curating the right resources to be successful is crucial. Done in the right way, patient education can help create a much more efficient practice for a physician and can help build communities focused on health creation. Dr. Sachin Patel implemented a personality assessment tool (DiSC) for each of his patients and team members to individualize the approach even farther, and I expect to see more of this innovation in personalized medicine.

QUESTION: *What information do you find yourself repeating to patients?*

ACTION: *Go to goevomed.com/calculator and take the test to see how much time you could save with an autoresponder.*

CHAPTER SEVEN

INCREASING YOUR EFFICIENCY

"Modern technology has become a total phenomenon for civilization, the defining force of a new social order in which efficiency is no longer an option but a necessity imposed on all human activity."

———JACQUES ELLUL

W HEN DR. DEBORAH MATTHEWS shifted her practice from primary care to functional medicine, she was okay with making less money in the short term as she established a viable practice she was passionate about. Though the practice became quite busy, it wasn't long before she noticed that the structure wasn't working as well as she wanted.

At the core, being busy doesn't equal being successful.

Dr. Matthews couldn't possibly schedule enough patients for sixty- or ninety-minute appointments for the practice to make any money, and she didn't have time to be a real entrepreneur because she was the one delivering all the care. Sound familiar? It's a common dilemma in functional medicine. Dr. Matthews felt she had two choices: push through and try to make it work, or decide that entrepreneurship wasn't for her and throw in the towel, taking a staff position instead.

Although this might be obvious to anyone in the industry, the recent IFM survey quantified this topic for the first time in 2016. On average, a functional medicine doctor sees 7.4 patients per day, whereas a typical primary care physician sees nineteen people. This is a problem for two main reasons. If the price point is high, it makes the doctor's care out of reach to anyone beyond the "very rich, very sick, or very green." If the price point is reasonable, it makes it hard for the doctor to make enough money to keep the practice doors open. What if we could increase the number of people seen each day and actually increase the quality of care at the same time? Best practices are emerging that make this possible.

Looking at these numbers, it seems the average functional doctor would need to see twelve patients per day, both to bring care to more of their community and earn more money than they would practicing primary care or family medicine. When doctors realize they can make more money with functional medicine than primary care, the floodgates will open.

I know this can be an uncomfortable topic for the functional medicine community, most of whom are practicing this medicine for reasons of clinical integrity, rather than financial gain. My training as an economist tells me that prices and profits send signals into the market, and so perhaps reframing the argument from personal enrichment to catalyzing a movement will make practice success more palatable for the current functional practices.

The role of the functional medicine doctor is multifaceted: doctor, educator, coach, teacher, and business owner. Dr. Matthews loved the excitement and empowerment of functional medicine but couldn't possibly do it all by herself. She worked with one of Evolution of Medicine's recommended partners, Freedom Practice Coaching, who analyzed her business and decided that the first priority was efficiency. Her practice was still within the structure of mainstream medicine, which held her back from seeing enough patients. Doctors caught between these two worlds of functional and conventional medicine need to find the resources and scalable technology for seamless communication. The potential for growth lies with three components: group office visits, creating provider teams, and better use of technology.

Functional medicine needs to massively improve its efficiency if it is going to become the standard of care. Efficient practices enable physicians to see more patients, yet each patient gets more time and attention from the team of providers. These teams can educate and empower patients in organized and automated ways that are also personal and relevant. This allow physicians to accept a steady number of new incoming patients, and the goal is to effectively reduce the dependence on doctors by providing empowerment, resources, and tools for health creation.

Let's first look at group structures, both for education as well as for clinical care.

Working with patients in groups is a really obvious way to improve efficiency. Not only do groups solve the resource constraint problem, but they also offer support, accountability, and patient education, and they promote participation. This maximizes the clinical efficacy at no extra cost.

Dr. Shilpa Saxena, a family physician in Lutz, Florida, started organizing group visits out of necessity. The other attending physician was out on maternity leave, and Dr. Saxena needed a way to meet with all of the patients. Within the group visit, she's able to see sixteen people at the same time and bill each person's insurance for a shared appointment. During that time, typically ninety minutes, there is a group education segment, and then a conversation facilitated by a second provider, often a nonbillable provider like a health coach or nutritionist. Meanwhile, the patients meet with Dr. Saxena to answer any specific questions about medication, supplements, and so on. We are seeing that best practices can include patients with similar complaints, but in functional medicine that can be a range of diagnoses due to common root causes. There are a few logistical and privacy issues to work out before you start doing it, but it is becoming a more and more accepted practice.

Shared appointments are an extension of an excellent idea that's been around for a while. The American Heart Association organizes groups for cardiovascular patients who have had heart attacks. Functional medicine seeks to empower patients within this group context. As with Dr. Saxena's practice, shared appointments can typically be billed on insurance. Other organizations are using the power of groups to bring this medicine to the underserved, and it is working so well that an article in the *New York Times* in May 2016 shared that "Group Doctor Visits Gain Ground," and some have even asked if this is the future of medicine.

Outside the strictly clinical realm, innovation is happening in functional medicine practice around the country as physician entrepreneurs look to solve this complex efficiency problem. One of the main reasons we loved having Freedom Practice Coaching, led by Dr. Charles Webb, as a sponsor of the Forum is the innovation they deliver in group approaches throughout their clinic model. It starts in new patient lead flow with their signature "community dinner talks" and continues with group education classes in the practice and even goes so far as hosting supermarket tours, showing practice members how to shop healthily in their local grocer. Talk about a remarkable experience!

Dr. Sachin Patel recently organized a cooking event for twenty patients. He kept hearing them complain they didn't have time to cook the healthy meals his program was recommending, or they didn't know what to make, so he ordered the ingredients and delivered them to a commercial kitchen, where participants worked with a chef and nutritionist to cook twenty meals in bulk. At the end of the ninety minutes, each person had made one dish that served twenty people, and each went home with a week's worth of healthy, varied meals, packed in neat Tupperware containers. All your food for one week in ninety minutes, plus nineteen new friends and new cooking skills. That smells like the future of medicine to me.

Hosting a walking group that meets weekly at the office is an easy way to engage with patients outside of appointments and promote health creation. Organizing meet-ups for patients with similar concerns helps everyone learn the same information without needing to meet with each person separately. If you add the community aspect to any healthy behavior like walking, you get a synergistic value proposition.

Group activities are central to functional medicine, where social relationships are considered an aspect of overall health. Introducing people to each other and creating new relationships can reduce costs, make discounted care more accessible, and add value to the patient experience. It goes above and beyond regular check-ups, and relates to Dr. George Slavich's research at the UCLA Stress Lab, where feeling connected is a better predictor of good health outcomes than exercising, eating healthily, or not smoking.

The next component of efficient practices is working with synergistic providers. In Dr. Frank Lipman's practice in New York, there are two doctors and seven health coaches. The old model assumed that the majority of the work had to be done by doctors, but this isn't true or particularly efficient. In order to run smoothly, functional medicine practices need to properly delegate responsibilities to other providers or community members. When working with a health coach, that could mean that patients who are booked for ninety-minute appointments spend thirty minutes with a doctor and an hour with the health coach. Patients receive the same value, and the physician-led team can see more patients each day.

Dr. Dean Ornish's program for heart disease uses a team of six providers working together, as well as group structures. In that system, out of the seventy-two hours of care provided for the patient, only an hour or two at the most is physician driven. The nurse case manager, stress reduction specialist, exercise physiologist, registered dietitian, and group facilitator do the majority of the heavy lifting, empowering the behavior change necessary to achieve the incredible results the program is known for.

At Parsley Health all the health coaching happens through a HIPAA-compliant video platform. Although the coaches don't work in the office itself, they are still an integral part of the team. Dr. Berzin designed Parsley as a medical practice that works to meet patients where they are. That includes organizing farm-to-table dinners, events at yoga studios, meditation workshops, and discussions on optimizing workplace health and food as medicine for its members. This brings Parsley Health into the community and helps bring the community into the fold of Parsley Health, and it makes my job so much easier to showcase examples of clinics really doing it right.

Speaking of clinics doing it right, the third place where we can add efficiency to the practice of functional medicine is with the use of effective technologies to scale and automate care. Dr. Berzin believes healthcare should be like your iPhone: go everywhere with you, be easy to use, and work efficiently. Healthcare is often in the dark ages when it comes to tech. Patients wait on hold for administrative assistants to pull records, scramble to find fax machines, and don't always have easy access to lab records. In an interview with the Functional Forum, Dr. Berzin said, "I believe people should own their data, they should be able to schedule online, they should be able to e-mail with their doctor, [and] they should be able to communicate in a modern way." She also believes physicians should be using available technologies to run their practices more efficiently. Some of the innovative ways Parsley is doing that include not having a phone number or a front desk. Communication is all done through e-mail or the patient EMR portal and that saves overhead, as she doesn't need a receptionist. Patient members enroll on the website and fill out many of the intake forms online before coming in for the first appointment.

When we started the Functional Forum, we realized much of this and so decided to only take sponsors whose products and services would rapidly increase the efficiency of Functional Medicine. In the next few paragraphs I will share some of the most inefficient areas of practicing functional medicine and share some of the best in category technology resources to solve those problems. We even have a podcast series called "The Future of Patient Compliance," where my partner Gabe Hoffman and I interview the founders of each technology to talk about this exact process. To see which of these technologies could be a fit, feel free to fill out our technology quiz at www.goevomed.com or schedule a free concierge call.

1. THE LENGTHY INTAKE

The most time-intensive aspect of functional medicine is the intake process. The IFM study released in 2016 showed that the majority of functional medicine doctors take more than sixty minutes—many took more than ninety minutes—for that initial appointment with a new patient. It's time-consuming because there are a lot of questions, which need to be fitted into a timeline and matrix. Some practitioners even admitted to not doing it thoroughly enough, despite seeing the value of it.

LivingMatrix is a technology that digitizes, automates, and visualizes the functional medicine matrix. Instead of sitting with a doctor and going over questions, a patient is sent an e-mail ahead of the appointment and asked to fill out a questionnaire online. The answers automatically populate the timeline and matrix, determining antecedents, triggers, and mediators. This radically reduces the amount of time it takes to do the intake, and allows the doctor to act like an editor instead of a scribe. It can also allow a doctor to review the information before seeing a patient, which gives them more time to formulate follow-up questions and consider options for care. LivingMatrix allows practitioners to add 1.3 people per day (from 7.4 to 8.7), can be integrated with Electronic Medical Records (EMR), and means that all members of the care team can review it and communicate relevant information.

2. NAVIGATING LAB TESTS

Another area of functional medicine that can be inefficient is the running of labs. Just think to yourself for a moment how much time is spent running the labs, interpreting the labs, having the blood drawn, and tracking down the patients. It can be a nightmare.

That is why we were thrilled to come across IGGBO, the "Uber for Phlebotomists." This startup is making waves (and attracting serious investors) by connecting labs, patients, doctors, and phlebotomists in a seamless technology platform. So, imagine that instead of having patients come back in for blood draws, you can send an "Iggy" or mobile phlebotomist to your patients' home or office. This takes compliance for lab tests from near 60% to over 98%, and given the percentage of medical decisions that are made from a drop of blood, this is a critical efficiency.

3. PROFESSIONAL SUPPLEMENTS

For any clinic shifting to functional medicine, one of the most unsavory parts is working out how to be truly empathetic with patients about supplementation. There are significant quality challenges with consumer-facing supplement brands you might find in Walmart or GNC, and the professional supplement world (there are 200+ brands that sell only through providers) has been somewhat thrown into disarray by the Internet, specifically Amazon undercutting the traditional markup made by practitioners. Earlier in the book, I referred to the new era as Functional Medicine 2.0. In my opinion, in Functional Medicine 3.0, when it is the standard of care, it will not be okay for doctors to make money from supplement sales, but we currently find ourselves in the "space between stories" and so we recommend a service that allows you total brand flexibility and a great technology platform to maximize retention and compliance.

With Fullscript, physicians can e-prescribe supplements to patients, without having to carry a massive amount of inventory in an office or warehouse. They offer integrated online and offline inventory so patients can try a probiotic given to them at an appointment and simply refill it through their doctor without having to visit the office. This ongoing communication portal allows doctors to make recommendations and monitor what patients are taking. This is so much more efficient for patients and practitioners, who don't need to keep inventory in stock and can keep overhead costs low. This capital can then be put toward new patient acquisition, which should be a priority for new practices.

4. REAL TIME COMMUNICATION

If there is one area where we can see the biggest impact of technology on efficiency it is communication, not only between providers and their patients, but also provider teams. Medical communication has so many massive inefficiencies, it isn't difficult to find a way to make a big impact.

Dr. Stephanie Daniel increased her practice's efficiency by 40% when she started using MDHQ, an EMR created specifically for functional medicine. I've heard plenty of horror stories of efficiency plummeting while practices learn how to incorporate EMRs, but over time, there are big efficiency gains with proper workflow integration. Used correctly, they organize communication efficiently between all the stakeholders. For Dr. Daniel's office, this was a huge gain. When she added telemedicine, she could conference with her patients remotely, which patients said fit in better with their schedules.

Telemedicine allows patients and physicians to conduct follow-up appointments from their respective homes or offices. In certain areas, the supply of functional medicine practitioners hasn't met the demand, so doctors use telemedicine to meet with patients who live farther away. It offers massive increases in efficiency for patients, who no longer need to take time off work to see their physician, as well as doctors, who no longer need a large office with lots of staff. Zoom has a HIPAA-compliant service that works quite well, but there is a range of different providers with different features and benefits.

5. BEHAVIOR CHANGE

There are a multitude of apps and platforms created for patients to track their behavior between appointments, where health actually happens. Some of them even integrate with wearable devices and mobile phones to track nutrition, exercise, and sleep. Handwritten food diaries, traditionally important to functional medicine, were a wildly inefficient way of tracking nutrition. Patients could quit after two days, and the doctor wouldn't know until the follow-up appointment the next month...if the patient actually shows up, which is doubtful if they are feeling ashamed or embarrassed about not doing what they committed to. Technologies like MBODY360, NudgeCOACH, and Mymee allow healthcare professionals to track patients in real time between appointments and get a sense of their progress. This helps with accountability. Both physician and patient spend less time communicating information face-to-face at follow-up appointments, but they still have a greater sense of engagement and connection, and have a data stream that can be used to uncover hidden triggers.

NudgeCOACH started out as a consumer platform, and their data tells an interesting tale. Those with professional support were 3.3 times more likely to still be actively engaging with mobile health after 120 days, and they also lost an average of 4.5 times more weight over the first 120 days. This proves our assertion that functional medicine coaching and technology are among the three pillars of the future of chronic disease care.

As the adage goes, you can't improve what you don't measure, and for that reason I see this "quantified self" revolution driving massive demand for functional medicine in the next decade, as people look to improve the numbers of their trackers. However, tracking is the just the first step, and there are also technologies that can actually speed up the process of behavior change. One such technology is HeartMath, a heart rate variability system that you can send patients home with. Using the technology, they can train themselves through their mobile app to maintain or achieve lower levels of stress.

The truth is that, most likely, the best technologies to run a functional medicine practice have yet to be created, but with all of those mentioned above we have heard consistently good feedback from practitioners and see that all of the companies are dedicated to improving their product and integrating with other technologies.

Looking to the future, the most efficient practices will likely use a combination of the strategies mentioned in this chapter. You can see how you need a basic provider team to pull off the two-provider group visit model, and a health coach would be a great person to lead a cooking evening or walking group. Any way to infuse the power of community into the practice will add significant value to the patient and to the bottom line, as we are still in the early adopter phase and these are remarkable patient experiences. If you're not sure where to start with these different technologies, you can book a free Evolution of Medicine concierge call at our website, www.goevomed.com.

QUESTION: *What in your practice represents the most unbilled time?*

ACTION: *Take the practice development survey at goevomed.com.*

CHAPTER EIGHT

BUILDING YOUR COMMUNITY

"A community is a group of people bound together by gifts and stories."

— CHARLES EISENSTEIN

T HE FUNCTIONAL FORUM STARTED with the intention of sharing the stories and wisdom of physicians practicing functional medicine. The hope was that doctors who were interested in learning about functional medicine could watch the interviews and talks for free, while those who were already practicing could learn about best practices and technologies then connect with others. People could learn how to start or improve a functional medicine practice from those who had already been through it. With the interactive live format, the Functional Forum allowed physicians to be in the same "room" together, communicating and working toward solutions, without needing to leave their home or office. By partnering with technology companies, the two worlds could talk, interact, and figure out how to best serve each other's needs. Those online events led to in-person meet-ups, and there are now over two hundred around the world. The Functional Forum started by giving gifts and sharing stories, and grew into a community.

Marketing is essential to a viable functional medicine practice, but the old model doesn't work anymore. People's attention is spread over a much broader range of media sources than a decade ago, and so many of the strategies that worked over the last few decades no longer do.

From our experience, practices need to focus on building community, which will bring a consistent stream of new patients and help retain current ones. In this new world of marketing, doctors are co-creating the practice with their patients and audiences, but it will be successful only if their practices are already efficiently run.

As noted earlier, Dr. Pamela Wible started building her community of patients and co-providers before she even built her practice. Holding a town hall-style meeting, she asked patients what kind of practice would be of value to them, and how much they would be willing to pay for that service. She then built a practice around the needs and values of her community.

However, whereas the first part of community building is to build what your community wants, the second part is to grow the community by sharing gifts and stories with more and more people. The goal is not to preach to the choir—current patients—but to grow the congregation, so to speak. In order for functional medicine to be an effective solution for non-communicable disease, it needs to reach way more people. For physicians whose practices are already established, there are lots of ways to give gifts, tell stories, and connect with the greater community.

First things first, we need to connect with the people who are already interested or have the potential to be. In a recent interview Dr. Joe Tatta, a physical therapist, shared that more and more physical therapy locations around the country are looking for functional medicine practitioners. A functional medicine micropractice would be the perfect addition to a physical therapy or chiropractic practice, many of which already work toward creating health by engaging patients in participatory care.

Outside the traditional framework of healthcare, physicians can connect with like-minded communities already in existence, like CrossFit franchise owners, personal trainers, people who frequent farmers' markets, health food stores, and healthy restaurants. CrossFit locations are excellent places to reach out, because their culture encourages education and is already interested in clean eating and paleo concepts. A functional medicine physician can hold a Q&A at a CrossFit gym for members, or a discussion at a yoga studio on how yoga benefits the digestive system. They can partner with a personal trainer to run free seminars on nutrition for their clients. A spa could host a clinician for a wellness day for people to make their own all-natural beauty products and discuss how diet, sleep, and stress impact skin health. Practices could connect with people at farmers' markets, hold a cooking event at a health food store, or a farm-to-table dinner at a restaurant. Connecting and aligning with those who have shared interests can create opportunities to bring them into the practice. We call this presidential marketing, and armed with an autoresponder and a personal story, this could be a quick way to build the practice and community.

Brands like Lululemon are catching onto this phenomenon. They organize running groups that meet at their stores, which provides a place for people to connect over a shared interest, as well as branding and marketing for the store. The example provided earlier, of Dr. Sachin Patel's cooking classes for patients, can be expanded and a physician could partner with a nutritionist or the owner of a juice bar to host a similar event. If someone is running a micropractice and doesn't have a huge space to host meetings, partnering with restaurants, cafes, and community centers is a great way to meet people where they are without increasing overhead. By organizing and hosting free events, the barrier to entry is low, and it provides a lot of value for potential patients. Event space is not a priority for a micropractice, but as a practice establishes and grows, teaching kitchens and community spaces can be useful additions.

The goal is to share your story with the people who are the most likely to listen, and then give something of value to the listeners as a gift. Tapping into existing communities and providers who are already unified around health is one of the easiest ways to do this. Receiving referrals from other practitioners is another way to connect with other groups of people, and it's definitely the fastest way to grow your practice. Local yoga studios, chiropractors, acupuncturists, massage therapists, and gym or spa owners are all great people to get to know. In our Accelerator we have example letters you could use as the basis of your mailer to these community linchpins.

After you have converted the low hanging fruit it is time to access the communities who aren't necessarily interested in functional medicine or haven't seen its role in health creation. This is the next group of people to attract into your practice. To do this we need what we call "Conversion Engines," events or technologies that turn interested people into patients. There are a number of ways to do this, even if you are an introvert or not a public speaker. Again, we turn to Dr. Gladd as an example.

The first time Dr. Gladd and I met, we were both speaking at a conference called "Heal Thy Practice" in Long Beach, California in 2011. One evening at the conference, we were able to see a first release version of an upcoming film called *Escape Fire: The Fight to Rescue American Healthcare*, which, if you have yet to see, I can't recommend more highly. The film expertly showcases the problems in American medicine, including physician burnout, excessive cost, and perverse incentives, and also shares some exciting solutions, all based in this new medical paradigm. I have yet to meet someone who has seen that film and at the end of it isn't fired up about seeing a functional medicine provider...or becoming one!

Impressed by the film, Dr. Gladd organized a screening of it in his home town of Fort Wayne, Indiana. He spent a couple of months promoting it to his patient community and asked them to invite friends, and scheduled a Q&A afterwards with the head of a local hospital. The results were astounding: 200 attendees, and 64 new patients signed on the spot. This isn't a one-off, either, and it doesn't just work in Indiana. In 2014, Tom Blue was launching a concierge practice in Ridgefield, Connecticut and used the same strategy, this time flying in one of the stars of the film *Dr. Erin Martin* for the Q&A with the local doctor. Their concierge practice was $250 a month or $3,000 annually and more than 100 new patients signed up on the spot, representing over $400k in practice revenue. Make sure to have new patient forms ready to go!

Re-creating this strategy has become even easier now that technology companies like Tugg and Gathr have popped up. These sites make it easy for anyone to organize a screening of their favorite films at a local theater. In October 2015 we launched the Evolution of Medicine Film Festival, encouraging our practitioner community to book a screening of *Escape Fire* through Tugg.com. One of the reasons we love Tugg is that not only do they take care of all the admin like negotiating with the movie maker and the theater, but they also set up the event page for you to sell tickets and have "Tugg School" on their site to make it easier for you to sell the required number. Some practitioners even pre-purchased tickets to give out to influential community members or their best referring patients. This is the perfect example of a powerful gift and an even more powerful story, which can't help but lead to a strong community, with your practice at the center. By providing patient education in a new, engaging way, physicians can help people create health, while also introducing their own story in their functional medicine practice.

A film screening is just one example of an event that you can use to convert patients. If you are a good speaker and have refined your practice message, putting on speaking events can be a great way to attract new patients. First focus on finding opportunities where the community is already assembled. Local chapters of national organizations like Kiwanis or Lions are always looking for good speakers, but you might also look for opportunities at local businesses (lunch and learns!) or community centers. Once you are consistently good at "converting people" with your talk, then you can start to pay to put bums in seats.

Some of the most effective practice marketing systems we see use flyers or Facebook ads to fill local events with enticing topics like "Stress and Hormones: The True Cause of Belly Fat" (a Freedom Practice Coaching favorite), knowing that whatever they pay to get people there in marketing will be made back and more by the lifetime value of the patients who sign up. Bottom line: You have to know your numbers. One key asset you can use in these events is patients with success stories who will likely be only too happy to share.

Dr. Sachin Patel has mastered this system. He puts his events up on Eventbrite, which is a free platform that more and more people are using to source local events. He fills the free education events using Facebook ads, knowing exactly how much to spend to fill the room, and knowing that only his target market (women age 30-70 living within 10 miles of his practice) will see the ad.

By doing these events in the community, there is also the added benefit of introducing health-minded people to each other, which adds value to their lives at no extra cost to you. Do you remember the work of Dr. Slavich from the UCLA Stress Lab I referenced earlier in the book? Communities are a more powerful form of medicine than nutrition, exercise, and smoking cessation, and connecting people around healthy habits is crucial to good outcomes. Introducing them to new people, new ideas, and potential accountability partners combines patient education, efficiency, and marketing. This kind of marketing is often more in line with a physician's practice, as some feel uncomfortable with traditional methods. It's a synergistic scenario where everyone wins.

Physicians who run events need two things: an autoresponder and easy access to online scheduling for new patients. When we discussed the importance of the autoresponder for an efficient practice, we mentioned that it helps physicians tell the story of how they became interested in functional medicine, why they practice it, and what they offer. Both of the basic autoresponder softwares we recommend in our Accelerator will communicate seamlessly with Eventbrite. Community events are an excellent way to add potential new patients to the e-mail list. Now that they've attended a meet-up, seminar, or class and walked away with something of value—a gift, if you will—a physician can send them a follow-up e-mail thanking them for their interest, furthering the story of the practice, and offering a link to online scheduling. In this new marketing model, community building becomes a way to meet new clients and co-providers. Can you see how the whole system works together?

By having an autoresponder and a link to online scheduling, physicians can track conversion rates—the number of new e-mail addresses that convert into new patients and appointments. Patients often want to schedule appointments in the hours that offices are closed—before or after work. In fact, data from zocdoc.com states that the majority of patients book appointments between 6:00 pm and 9:00 am, when most practices are closed.

As I mentioned earlier, Dr. Berzin's practice, Parsley Health, doesn't have a phone number at all. Every new member is signed up through the website, and every subsequent appointment is set up via the EMR patient portal. Operating on a membership model, patients don't pay more if they have to book multiple appointments. The single appointment is a reflection of the old model of fee-for-service and acute disease. The membership model ensures a predictable monthly revenue, and that patients are committed to ongoing, participatory care. Getting to the root of chronic conditions takes time, and business models like Parsley Health reflect that.

A lot of practices that rely on scheduling over the phone miss out on tracking conversion rates, as front desks traditionally don't. For five years, my wife and I built websites for doctors, and most wanted to push people to the clinic's phone number. If you don't know how well your front desk is converting calls to patients, you can't determine or plan for growth. The Evolution of Medicine's Accelerator program outlines how practices can train front desk associates to find out how a patient learned about the practice, engage them before they come in, and obtain necessary and relevant information to individualize their care.

Practices need systems in place for focused marketing and conversion. There's a cost for each new patient acquisition—the time it took to set up the autoresponder, host the event, and associated costs. By knowing how many new patients come in each week or month through these marketing strategies, a physician can figure out the cost of each new patient acquisition and compare it to the lifetime value of the patient.

The most effective practitioners know the cost and value.

Although 75% of practices are cash-based, according to an IFM survey, most had yet to wrap their heads around the realities of operating a business. Businesses need to pay to acquire and retain new clients, and they need to figure out how to do so in a way that is cost-effective. There is an economic incentive to growing a cash-based practice. Starting small, with free events and small numbers of audiences, and scaling up as the business grows is a great way to do this. As more people sign up, you can expand the scope of your talks and events.

Some patients might come in right away, and others won't make an appointment until they or someone they know gets sick. Others might not even attend an event but hear about the practice through an employee, a current patient, or someone who did attend an event. Taking note of how people find the practice is crucial to figuring out what strategies are working and are cost-effective.

Technology is a great way to focus marketing, but one word of warning. In Functional Medicine 1.0 the best way to market your practice was to be seen as an expert, meaning that most early adopter doctors went the way of Internet marketing: write a book, build an e-mail list, become a health celebrity.

That was fine at the start, but the problem is that it isn't a sustainable model. Think about Twitter. Does it make sense to build a big Twitter following if 99.9% of users are not within twenty miles of your practice? Also, we can't have 100,000 health celebrities. We need new models of practice marketing that are sustainable and focus on bringing the local community together.

All of these methods and approaches are different from traditional marketing, because if we want to create health—as opposed to treat disease—we need to do very different things. A disease-management system depends on people being ill in order for them to come in, and it relies on the $6 billion marketing budget of the pharmaceutical companies to tell the population to "ask your doctor if _____ might be right for you." One of the biggest traps doctors fall into when they make the switch is to assume that will carry on.

Functional medicine aims to end disease, in a certain way putting itself out of business, and relies on patients to participate in the process. Connecting with people who are already working toward creating health means supporting them on that journey and helping them prevent future illness. The best systems we've seen in marketing are these conversion events— dinner talks or other venues, where a doctor gets people in the room in order to tell a focused story of functional medicine and the value that it provides for people's lives.

The Evolution of Medicine Practice Accelerator has resources and assets to help physicians plan, organize, and track events and marketing opportunities. There are examples of great talks, ideas for film screenings, tutorials on how to get people in the room, and tips on how to convert attendees into patients. We're not aiming to cultivate a generation of celebrity doctors—we're aiming for physicians to get in front of people in their community and tell stories of health creation. We're aiming for effective practices that are reproducible by any doctor in any community around the world.

QUESTION: *What gifts could you give and stories could you tell to build your community?*

ACTION: *Make a list of existing communities you'd like to connect with.*

CHAPTER NINE

BECOMING AN EVANGELIST

"Never doubt that a small group of thoughtful, committed citizens can change the world; indeed, it's the only thing that ever has."

———MARGARET MEAD

THE FINAL STAGE OF the hero's journey is becoming an evangelist. Once you go through the final test of building a successful micropractice, you're at the point where you can be an evangelist for the movement. The main reason for creating an efficient micropractice is to free up the physician's time and engage the patient in participatory care. Now that we have this extra time with the new business model, let's use it to do something really powerful and awesome. Luckily, there are countless ways to help. Some hold community events, write blogs, start podcasts, and volunteer their time. Others become teachers, build empires, or create television shows. There are opportunities for everyone to become an evangelist for functional medicine, inspiring more patients and doctors to join the evolution in their own way.

Since starting his own micropractice, Dr. Jeffrey Gladd works no more than three days per week in the office, picks his kids up from school, coaches recreational sports teams, and hasn't worked a Friday in six years. His personal life and work are well-balanced, he's more in love with his career than ever, and he's the first to tell people about it. "I couldn't be happier in practicing medicine," he said in a Functional Forum interview. He added that his kids are even interested in taking the path, because they see how much he enjoys it.

He started out wanting to lose fifty pounds and regain his health so he could help his patients do the same. Now, he has a successfully functioning practice, and he says that every new patient leads to a few more, as family members and friends remark on the quality of care. Dr. Gladd mentors and consults with doctors looking to start functional medicine practices, and he teaches at the University of Arizona, George Washington University, and the Integrated Health Symposium in New York. He's an advocate of digital health platforms, having started Mytavin.com to help patients track prescriptions and symptoms of drug-induced nutrient depletion.

Dr. Gladd's success helps him prove to curious doctors that they can create a viable practice in their own community. He's spreading the message of functional medicine to physicians, patients, and the tech industry. Even though his first integrative medicine practice in a hospital was shut down, he has shown through his own practice in Indiana that functional medicine is possible in communities around the world. The evangelism phase will look different depending on the goals of practitioners.

For doctors like Dr. Robin Berzin, spreading the message of functional medicine means opening up new clinics. During the summer of 2016, merely a year and a half after opening the first Parsley Health in New York, Dr. Berzin is establishing the second Parsley Health in Los Angeles, with plans for another branch in San Francisco. Dr. Berzin's low-overhead membership model is easily reproducible, with massive opportunities for growth. As a patient of Dr. Berzin, I can attest to how remarkable that practice is. With the sea change in health care, there are incredible opportunities for new models and franchises.

In the UK, Dr. Rangan Chatterjee hosts BBC One's "Doctor in the House," which follows him as he works closely with families for a month at a time. The first season aired in November 2015, and four million UK viewers (and millions more around the world) watched as he coached people through healthy food choices, good sleep habits, stress management, and work routines. What he found was that people are confused. With so many claims and studies that seem to change every minute, conflicting health information made lifestyle changes difficult. The BBC One program shows that health creation takes time and participation. Rather than ten-minute visits with a specialized practitioner, Dr. Chatterjee's approach is hands-on and geared toward generalized medicine. Over the course of a month, his work with patients has reversed cases of type 2 diabetes, opioid addiction, eczema, and hormone imbalances. After an epic first season, the show has been confirmed for a second season in 2017.

Another recognizable figurehead of functional medicine is Dr. Mark Hyman, who runs a practice in Lenox, Massachusetts and is now the director of the Cleveland Clinic Center for Functional Medicine. He's often a guest on television shows and writes columns for a number of high-profile outlets, and many are familiar with Dr. Mark Hyman's best-selling books, such as *The Blood Sugar Solution: 10 Day Detox Diet,* and *Eat Fat, Get Thin.* Publishing articles and books offers an immense amount of value to patients and people looking to create health. This way, they can access the information at any time and use it as a resource on their journey. For physicians, books are excellent marketing tools and can be used to schedule appearances on local and national radio and television programs. We aren't quite at *peak* health celebrity, but we are close.

Dr. Robynne Chutkan has published multiple books, *The Bloat Cure, The Microbiome Solution* and *GutBliss*, and runs a wildly successful blog regarding GI research. Dr. Kelly Brogan's book,

A Mind of Your Own, discusses how depression in women is a symptom that can be cured by healing the body. Released in March 2016, it quickly became a *New York Times* bestseller. For doctors who are daunted by the prospect of writing a book, or don't have the time, Book in a Box has created a process to help people turn ideas into books (and if you're enjoying this book, that's how this was made—goevomed.com/bookinabox).

Other doctors who are spreading the word through innovative portals include Dr. Lissa Rankin, host of *The Fear Cure* on PBS, which raises money for public television. Dr. Steven Masley's book, *The 30 Day Heart Tune Up*, was one of the most successful fundraising drives for PBS in its history, connecting with millions of viewers. Some physicians write columns and articles for venues like the *New York Times*. Others have started podcasts to share their story, interview patients and other physicians, and connect with listeners around the world. There are physicians who have their own YouTube channel, and post short, focused talks on current events in medicine and aspects of health creation. These podcasts, videos, articles, and books are evidence of a physician's work and knowledge. It serves to further patient education and provides content that can be accessed by almost anyone, almost anywhere. With the rise of digital media, there are countless ways for clinicians to deliver to huge audiences worldwide. It helps spread the sphere of influence.

Some of the best practices we have seen are digital platforms that lead to in-person meet-ups and community events. There seems to be a great synergy between the two and it is questionable whether purely digital health relationships replicate the value of physical community.

However, we must take a moment to honor those who have been on the front lines treating patients week in and week out, sometimes for decades. We sometimes have a tendency to think the only way to scale one's impact is through celebrity, but the network effects of inspiring, consistent, and effective practices have powerful impact, beyond the patients or members of the practices and into the communities where they reside.

This is unquestionably a movement.

Functional Medicine 1.0 saw the rise of figureheads who have become celebrities for the cause. This gave us the momentum we needed to inform the mainstream. Functional Medicine 2.0 is about scalable, reproducible models of functional medicine and making sure there are more practices popping up around the world to meet this growing demand.

With high and rising rates of chronic disease, we can't wait seventeen years for new science to find its way into clinical practice. In what other industry and in what other time in history was there the potential to use today's science and information to build a remarkably improved practice, and create a business that could serve your community and your family for generations? That is the opportunity in front of you.

QUESTION: *If you practiced only three days a week, what would you spend the rest of your time doing?*

ACTION: *Schedule a concierge call at goevomed.com.*

THE END OF CHRONIC DISEASE

CHRONIC DISEASE IS ONE of the biggest issues currently facing humankind. It isn't lost on me, as someone who has been in this field almost my whole life, that there are many powerful players who benefit from the proliferation of chronic disease. Large medical stakeholders like pharmaceutical companies, insurance companies, and hospitals typically have a fiduciary responsibility to shareholders to maximize profits, leading to a suboptimal environment for these changes to occur. When I had the opportunity to ask Sir Richard Branson about taking on these established players, his view is that in order to take them on, your product or service has to be significantly better than the established players. I think it's clear from this book that, in this case, we are in good shape, and as I said in the very first Functional Forum, "We need to start acting like we're winning, and stop acting like we're losing."

My hope is that some of the concepts in this book will form the engine for medical transformation, even if that solution doesn't end up looking like the network of physician-owned community micropractices we currently envision.

Our vision depends on your success.

We are betting on the physician entrepreneur.

The future of functional medicine, and all medicine, might end up looking more like Uber or CrossFit, depending on the entrepreneurial appetite of doctors in each country as it scales up. Who will be the owners, and who will be the workers? Only time will tell.

However, I think it's just as important *how* we end chronic disease as whether we end it at all. Elegant medical solutions based in systems thinking, root cause resolution, therapeutic relationships, and patient empowerment are remarkable enough just for the patient. But a whole score of good things occur for the family, the physician, and the practice with each success as well. Beyond that, the real value occurs when that same thinking is then applied to other areas of one's life, relationships, and circumstances. I'll even dare to go as far as to say that the biggest value to society would be seeing this thinking applied to large, systemic issues like the environment, social policy, criminal justice, the economy and even the heart of politics—the subject for my second book.

This concept showcases a phenomenon that caused me to change my career eleven years ago: *positive externalities*. Externalities are an economics term describing the extra cost or benefit delivered to others that are unaccounted for in any transaction. The toxins I mentioned in Chapter 2 are often cited as a classic example of a negative externality, but obvious positive externalities are harder to pinpoint.

In my opinion, the positive externalities generated by the successful delivery of this medicine at scale have the power to outweigh the huge swathes of negative externalities delivered by the current system. Think about the ripple effects of a family empowered by a child's recovery, or the community around an adult going through his or her own hero's journey to reverse chronic disease. We are more interconnected than we think, and as greater numbers of people go through these transformational experiences, the benefits accrue to a much larger population than we might imagine.

We are living in a time of great transition. Wherever you are reading this, it's likely that there are plenty of local or national indicators that things aren't looking all that rosy—politically, economically, or socially. We are in what Charles Eisenstein calls "a space between stories" in his masterful work *The More Beautiful World our Hearts Know is Possible* (which is my top book suggestion for almost anyone I meet). The old story of control, force, and separation—a hallmark of the first era of medicine—is definitely on its way out, but we are not quite ready for the new story of community, empathy, and interdependence. Technology, the great supposed savior of the old story, cannot provide complete solutions to problems in this realm, but it can certainly accelerate the process toward success or failure.

The success of businesses and movements rooted in the new story over the last decade—from organic food to the sharing economy—are sending a signal to the market that systems thinking, peer-to-peer support, and all aspects of community are here to stay. This is the backbone of the new economy.

Functional medicine is rooted in the new story. My hope is that as the medical systems of the world align themselves to functional medicine and millions of patients go through this transformative hero's journey, it will thrust humankind into the new story, providing new answers and sustainable solutions to some of humankind's biggest problems.

ACKNOWLEDGEMENTS

T HERE ARE SO MANY people who played an important
role in the creation of this book and the founding of this
movement, and have been of huge support, inspiration, and
influence throughout the first part of my journey—including many people, I am sure, whom I will fail to mention in
this section.

First and foremost I would like to thank my parents for instill-
ing in me the direction of a life of purpose. Both of them
followed their callings and everyone who knows them around
the world always tells me how lucky I was to be born to such
incredible humans.

They also inadvertently thrust me into this world of functional medicine, as the doctor who C-sectioned me out of my
mother's womb in Loveland, Colorado in 1980 was one of the
founding members of the American Holistic Medical Association. Growing up in England and South Africa, I was the
only kid whose school nurse had to call the parents before
administering antibiotics, and who knew what a chiropractor
was. As the years tick by and science evolves, I am increasingly
grateful for their foresight.

Thanks to my mentor on the HSBC trading desk who did me a huge favor by getting drunk at his leaving party and telling me to "not waste my life sitting behind the same desk for thirty years" like he had.

A special thanks to two incredible mentors who I wouldn't have got this far without, Chuck Reddick for teaching me how to listen to doctors, and Seth Godin for teaching me about the importance of earning attention and trust and serendipitously scheduling an impresario training at a critical juncture in the journey.

Thanks to all the thousands of heroic doctors, practitioners, friends, and entrepreneurs I've met in the eleven years since I started down this path, some of whose stories you will find in this book and many who have been in the right place at the right time to provide encouragement, insight, and honesty needed for this book to be birthed. You know who you are!

Many of the ideas in this book have crystallized after long conversations with great friends I like to refer to as the "Leaders of the New School" like Dr. Jeffrey Gladd, Dr. Kelly Brogan, Dr. Rangan Chatterjee, Dr. Robin Berzin, Dr. Alejandra Carrasco, Dr. Sachin Patel, and "Dr." Tom Blue. This book wouldn't be possible without them on the front lines innovating on truly effective patient care models. I must also give a shout out to Erik Goldman for giving me my first opportunity to speak to hundreds of doctors at once from his stage.

My business partner, Gabe Hoffman, deserves much credit as we have built this movement together over the last three years, and the whole EvoMed team, especially Uli, Anthony, Melanie, Drew, and Anne. Legends all!

Lastly, there is one person I haven't thanked who has operated as the second half of my brain for over a decade. My wife Rachel is one of the most supportive and loving people I've ever known. Entrepreneurship can be a fundamentally selfish endeavor, and I'll always be grateful to her for letting me go first.

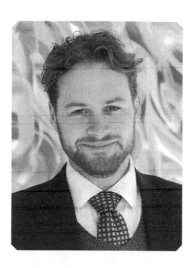

ABOUT THE AUTHOR

WITH THE SOUL OF an advocate and the mind of an entrepreneur, JAMES MASKELL has spent the past decade sparking debate and encouraging a shift away from conventional Western medicine and toward a wellness-centered, functional medicine model—starting with the doctors themselves. To that end, he created Functional Forum, the world's largest integrative medicine conference with record-setting participation online and growing physician communities around the world. He's also the founder of the Evolution of Medicine, a community e-commerce platform that provides highly curated and customized resources, tools, products, and services, making it easier and more affordable for conventional doctors to embark on a new way of managing healthcare.

An in-demand speaker and lively impresario, with a broad and thriving network in the functional medicine space, James lectures internationally and has been featured on TEDMED, Huffpost Live, TEDx and more, and is a contributor to Huffington Post, KevinMD, thedoctorblog, and MindBodyGreen. He serves on the faculty of George Washington University's Metabolic Medicine Institute and speaks regularly on the integrative medicine conference circuit. He graduated with honors from University of Nottingham with a degree in health economics.

He lives in Venice Beach, California, with his wife and daughter.

82754260R00086

Made in the USA
Middletown, DE
05 August 2018